Royal College of Obstetricians and Gynaecologists

Basic Practical Skills in Obstetrics and Gynaecology

Participant Manual

WITHDRAWN

Second edition of

Basic Surgical Skills

Supported by

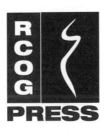

ETHICON   **RCOG PRESS**

Supported by

COVIDIEN
positive results for life

ISBN 978-1-904752-51-6

Published by the RCOG Press at the
Royal College of Obstetricians and Gynaecologists
27 Sussex Place, Regent's Park
London NW1 4RG

Registered Charity No. 213280

RCOG Press Editor: Jane Moody
Index: Liza Furnival, Medical Indexing Ltd
Design & typesetting: Karl Harrington, FiSH Books
Printed by Chris Fowler International, London, UK

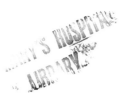

Contents

Basic Practical Skills in Obstetrics and Gynaecology Working Group

Rina Agrawal MRCOG

Sabaratnam Arulkumaran FRCOG, President, RCOG

Louise Ashelby MRCOG

Maggie Blott FRCOG, Vice President, Education, RCOG

Andrew Loughney MRCOG

Sandeep Mane MRCOG

Brenda Nathanson, Education Development Officer, RCOG

Manjit Obhrai FRCOG

Mark Roberts MRCOG

Clive Spence-Jones FRCOG

Introduction to the course

This handbook has been prepared for participants on the Royal College of Obstetricians and Gynaecologists' Basic Practical Skills in Obstetrics and Gynaecology course. The course has been designed to introduce trainees to safe surgical techniques and obstetric clinical skills in a structured workshop environment.

It is a requirement that this course is completed during ST1/2 before trainees move to ST3. The course consists of three modules and covers basic surgical skills and basic skills in obstetrics. In each module, the importance of sound knowledge of anatomy, the correct development of tissue planes, the appropriate use of traction and counter-traction, the need to obtain meticulous haemostasis and the importance of gentle tissue handling will be emphasised. In addition, the trainees will be taken through basic obstetrics skills and will have the opportunity to practice these skills under direct supervision.

The course runs from a number of approved regional centres and is standardised to ensure that common objectives, content structure and assessment methods are followed. The contents of the course do not represent the only safe way to perform a procedure but endeavour to give trainees one safe approach to common obstetric and gynaecological procedures. There is an emphasis on acquiring practical skills.

Each course will include:

■ considerable hands-on practical experience

■ high tutor to participant ratio

■ course handbook and CD-ROM

■ performance assessment with feedback to identify strengths and weaknesses.

Courses are offered under the aegis of the Royal College of Obstetricians and Gynaecologists and are held both at the College and locally to maximise convenience and reduce costs. The centres and their facilities selected for surgical and obstetric skills training have been approved by the College and are directed by RCOG-approved preceptors.

It is hoped that this course will be a valuable early step in building safe and sound surgical and obstetric skills. It should be instructive, educational and fun. We hope that you will find the course both useful and enjoyable and that it provides you with a firm foundation for your future career in obstetrics and gynaecology.

I am grateful to the previous Basic Surgical Skills Working Group, under the Chairmanship of Professor Garry, on which this new course has been based. I would also like to acknowledge the work of Mr Mark Roberts, Mr Andrew Loughney and Mr Sandeep Mane.

Maggie Blott FRCOG
Vice President, Education, Royal College of Obstetricians and Gynaecologists

Outline of the course

Day one

- Introduction to the course
- Principles of safe and effective surgery
- Theatre etiquette/correct gloving and gowning
- Theatre instruments and their use
- Specific instruments for use in obstetrics and gynaecology
- Handling instruments
- Knot tying
- Suturing
- Anatomy of anterior abdominal wall
- Surgical incisions into abdomen
- Opening and closing the abdomen
- Principles of haemostasis

Day two

- Anatomy of the pelvic floor and spontaneous vaginal birth
- **Scenario 1:** ventouse delivery, manual removal of placenta, episiotomy and repair, perineal tear
- **Scenario 2:** pudendal block and forceps, shoulder dystocia, postpartum haemorrhage
- **Scenario 3:** cardiotocograph interpretation, fetal blood sampling, caesarean section and documentation

Day three

- Endoscopic equipment: 'Meet the stack'
- Electrosurgery
- Principles of safe and effective hysteroscopy
- Laparoscopy and entry
- Demonstrations and practicals:

  Station 1: gynaecological examinations/pelvic swabs/smear taking/endometrial biopsy/intrauterine contraceptive device insertion

  Station 2: basic hysteroscopy/uterine evacuation

  Station 3: principles of closed laparoscopic entry

- Practical sessions: gynaecological examination/pelvic swabs/smear taking/ endometrial biopsy/intrauterine contraceptive devices and procedures; hysteroscopy/uterine evacuation; principles of safe laparoscopic entry

- Course review followed by free session for personal learning and revisit to stations

Module 1

Basic open general surgical techniques

Learning objectives

On completion of this module you will:

- understand the principles of safe surgery and theatre etiquette

- understand the importance of gentle handling of tissues and meticulous haemostasis

- understand that careful and sound technique is more important than speed

- demonstrate appropriate instrument handling

- demonstrate appropriate suturing and knotting techniques

- understand the importance of each member of the theatre team and treating all with respect.

Introduction

This module of the course is designed to teach you basic safe methods of performing simple surgical procedures and to allow you to perform and practise them using specifically designed tissue simulators and various jigs. We aim to provide you with an enjoyable hands-on experience and the opportunity to practise vital and fundamental techniques in an atmosphere less stressed than the operating theatre.

The module aims to introduce you to some of the skills you will require in your career. Complex manoeuvres will need to be assiduously practised, preferably under critical observation, so that you do not acquire bad habits. The aim of this course is to help you acquire good habits early in your career, as it is much harder to unlearn bad habits later in life. The techniques chosen for this course by the RCOG are simple and safe but we make no claim that these are the only simple techniques with proven safety. An advantage of the British system of training is that you will probably work for several surgeons in the course of your training, each of whom will show you individually preferred techniques from which you will be able to select those which suit your needs best. However, the techniques taught on this course have been standardised and are recommended for their simplicity and safety.

Preparation for the course

You should read this manual before attending the course. The course should be taken as early as possible in your surgical career and completed before entry into ST3.

Principles of safe surgery and good theatre etiquette

The theatre team

Teamwork is essential for effective surgery. It is essential that the surgeon acknowledges and values the contribution of each member of the team. All staff should be treated courteously. Surgeons should be particular about maintaining the highest standards and must ensure that their expectations are understood and that they are compatible with the goals of the other members of the team. The medical staff are complemented by nursing and ancillary staff who have the following roles:

- scrub nurse
  Prepares swabs, instruments, skin preparation and drapes and hands them over to the surgeon when required. The scrub nurse assists the surgeon by counting the instruments present at the end of the operation and checking that the instrument count is correct.

- assistant nurse (runner)
  Assists with swab count, opens packs and additional instruments and needles as required. Will often assist with positioning patient and applying diathermy plate. May assist with adjusting the stack system during laparoscopic procedures.

- operating department assistant

Responsible for assisting the anaesthetist during the induction of anaesthesia and with positioning the patient and maintaining equipment during the operation.

Preparation for surgery

An optimum surgical approach allows the operation to proceed with as little stress as possible to the patient, the surgeon and assisting theatre staff.

Patient positioning

When transferring the patient to the operating table, care must be taken to avoid injury to both the patient and the staff. The use of a slide saves lifting. Care must be taken to ensure that, when the patient is placed on the operating table, none of the skin is in contact with the metal parts of the table. This reduces the risk of electrical leakage to earth when diathermy is activated. Operate with the table at an appropriate height and with the patient in the correct position to provide the optimum view of the operative field. This will often be in a Trendelenberg 'head down' position so that bowel and omentum move away from the operative field of the pelvis, provided that there are few adhesions. Care should be taken that the patient is positioned so as to avoid her slipping off the operating table. The surgeon and assistants should avoid unknowingly resting on any part of the patient's body.

Ensure good views

Ensure that a clear view with good illumination is maintained throughout the operation and that there is adequate exposure. Always keep the operative field tidy with the minimum number of instruments in the wound.

Patient and staff safety

Check the integrity of instruments before use. This is especially important with electrical and endoscopic equipment. Sharp instruments should be handled in a way that reduces the risk of inadvertent injury, the blade of a knife should be guarded and the handle passed foremost, preferably via a kidney dish or suitable container. Patient safety as well as that of the theatre personnel remains the surgeon's responsibility. Always ensure that needles and blades are disposed of in a specific 'sharps' container.

Protective clothing and hand washing

Outdoor clothes should be removed and theatre scrubs and shoes worn. It is advised that a theatre hat, a mask and visor should be worn during all procedures. Hand washing is the single most important means of preventing the spread of infection. Areas most commonly missed when hands are washed are the thumbs, the backs of the hands, between the fingers and fingertips (Figure 1.1).

Hands should be washed before all procedures: when moving from patient to patient, after visiting the toilet, before handling food and when moving from a 'dirty' to a 'clean' task on the same patient. Hands must be washed even if gloves are worn.

The level of hand hygiene will also be determined by the activity or area of practice:

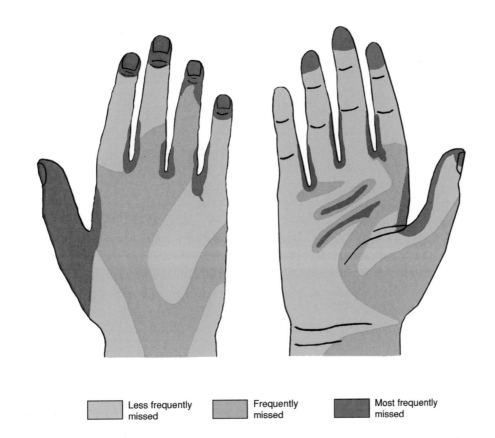

| Less frequently missed | Frequently missed | Most frequently missed |

Figure 1.1
Areas commonly missed during hand washing

Asepsis and hygiene

An antiseptic solution, such as Hibiscrub® (AstraZeneca), should be used prior to invasive procedures, in high-dependency areas and after attending patients in isolation with known transmissible conditions. Hand rubs are used to rapidly decontaminate visibly clean hands and between patient contact if hands are not contaminated with blood or organic matter. The alcohol content of the hand gel should be greater than 60%. All areas of the hands must be covered by the gel and hands must be rubbed together until all the gel has evaporated.

Surgical hand wash

■ Use an antiseptic solution such as Hibiscrub® (AstraZeneca), chlorhexidine or iodine; this is more effective than soap.

■ Remove all jewellery.

■ Cover cuts and abrasions with a waterproof dressing.

■ Wet hands before applying soap/antiseptic.

■ Lather well and rub hands together, paying particular attention to the tips of the fingers, the thumbs and the areas between the fingers.

■ Extend the wash to the arms as far as the elbows and rinse well afterwards.

■ Use a nail brush for 30 seconds on each hand, then rinse.

■ Wash a second time for 2 minutes – both hands up to the elbows, then rinse.

■ Wash a third time for 1 minute – both hands up to one-third away from elbow, then rinse with hands uppermost, allowing water to drain towards the elbows.

■ Dry your hands and arms using individual towels and blotting away all moisture.

Gown

Your gown should be put on by holding it in front of you and, as it unfolds, insert your arms into the sleeves. An assistant should pull the gown on from behind and tie the inside ties of the gown. A colleague who is scrubbed and gowned can assist you with the wrap-around tie.

Gloves

Gloves protect skin from contamination but only give minimal protection from sharps injuries. Gloves should be used for protection from exposure to blood/body fluids during procedures for all patients, including venepuncture, pelvic examination, wound management and surgery. Latex-free gloves should be available for those who have latex allergy.

> **Key features of the ideal glove**
>
> ■ It fits well and does not lose its shape.
>
> ■ It offers optimum sensitivity and durability.
>
> ■ It is powder-free, to reduce adhesions and allergy.
>
> ■ It contains low levels of latex protein.

Gloves are put on without touching the external surface of the gloves (closed glove technique). Having done this, adopt a 'scrub position' by holding your hands in front of you and being careful not to contaminate yourself before starting surgery.

Suture materials and needles

Suture characteristics

The ideal suture would consist of material which permits its use in any operation; the only variable being the size, as determined by the tensile strength. It should handle comfortably and naturally to the surgeon. The tissue reaction stimulated should be minimal and should not create an environment favourable to bacterial growth. The breaking strength should be high in a small calibre thread. A knot should hold securely without fraying or cutting. The material must be sterile. It should not shrink in tissues. It should be non-electrolytic, non-capillary, non-aller-genic and non-carcinogenic. Finally, after most operations the suture material should be absorbed with minimal tissue reaction after it has served its purpose.

No single type of suture material has all these properties and, therefore, no one suture material is suitable for all purposes. Besides, the requirement for wound support varies in different tissues for a few days for muscle, subcutaneous tissue and skin to weeks or months for fascia and tendon to long-term stability for vascular prosthesis.

Types of suture material

Suture materials are either absorbable or non-absorbable. Absorbable sutures offer temporary wound support over a period of time and thereafter are gradually absorbed either through a process of enzymatic reaction (catgut) or hydrolysis (synthetic materials). It is important to recognise that losing tensile strength and losing mass absorption are two separate events, because a suture may support the wound for only a very short time and yet be present as a foreign body for a long period afterwards. The ideal suture would be one which disappeared immediately after its work was complete but such a suture does not yet exist.

Non-absorbable sutures are not absorbed but some, especially those of biological origin, lose strength without any change in the mass of the suture material. Others gradually fragment over time. Yet other non-absorbable sutures, especially those of synthetic origin, never lose their tensile strength or change in mass following implantation.

Sutures can be subdivided into monofilament or multifilament. A monofilament suture is made of a single strand. It resists harbouring micro-organisms but has poor tying qualities. A multifilament suture consists of several filaments twisted or braided together. It is therefore easy to handle and ties secure knots.

A further classification is based in the origin of the raw material; it can either be from a biological source such as catgut or from man-made fibres. Sutures have been produced from a biological or natural source for many thousands of years. They tend to create greater tissue reaction than man-made sutures; the result can be localised irritation or even rejection. Another disadvantage is that factors present in the individual patient, such as infection and general health, can affect the rate at which enzymes attack and break down absorbable natural sutures. Man-made or synthetic sutures, on the other hand, are very predictable and elicit minimal tissue reaction. The most common man-made absorbable sutures are polymers of glycolide and lactin. Loss of tensile strength ranges from 10–14 days (rapid) to 28–30 days (medium), depending on the suture and coating used. For more prolonged tensile strength, polydioxanone monofilament may be used. The actual suture mass may take two to three times as long to be completely absorbed.

Suture selection

When repairing perineal lacerations after childbirth, prolonged tensile strength is not required but rapid absorption of foreign body may reduce infection risk and speed the healing process. Repair of fascia, such as the rectus sheath after suprapubic transverse abdominal incision, requires retention of suture tensile strength for a longer period. Abdominal skin incisions are commonly repaired with a subcuticular monofilament suture which is cosmetic and minimises risk of infection from skin flora drawn down the suture line. Absorbable subcuticular sutures should not be dyed for risk of leaving a visible residue. If a non-absorbable suture such as poly-propylene is used it is often removed after 5–7 days.

Selection of appropriate needles

Surgical eyeless needles are manufactured in a wide range of types, shapes, lengths and thicknesses. The choice of needle to be used depends on several factors such as:

- the requirements of the specific procedure
- the nature of the tissue being sutured
- the accessibility of the operative area
- the gauge of suture material being used
- the surgeon's preference.

Regardless of use, however, all surgical needles have three basic components; the point, the body and the swage (Figure 1.2).

The point depends on the needle type (see next section). The body of the needle usually has a flattened section where the needle can be grasped by the needle holder. In addition, some needles have longitudinal ribs on the surface which reduce rotational movement and ensure that the needle is held securely in the jaws of the needle holder. If the needle does not have a flattened section, then it should be grasped at a point approximately two-thirds of the needle length from the tip (Figure 1.3).

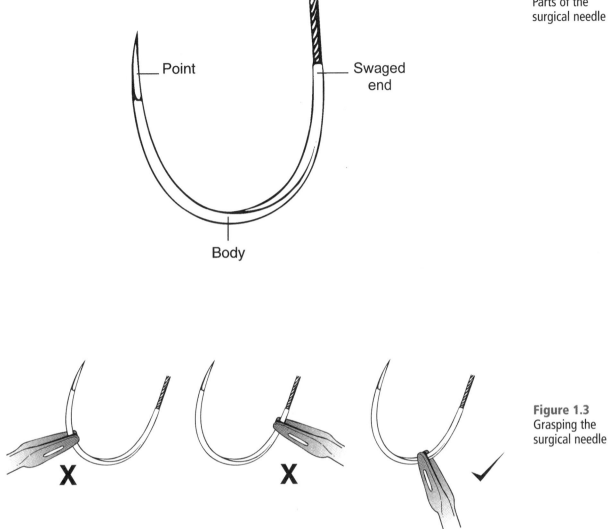

Figure 1.2
Parts of the
surgical needle

Figure 1.3
Grasping the
surgical needle

The majority of surgical needles used are eyeless; that is, they are already swaged to the suture material. This has many advantages, including reduced handling and preparation and less trauma to the tissue (an eyed needle has to carry a double strand which creates a larger hole and causes greater disruption to the tissue). A swaged (eyeless) needle has either a drilled hole or a channel at the end of the needle for insertion of the suture material. The drilled hole or the channel is closed round the needle in the swaging process. Needles are normally classified according to needle type. The two main categories are round-bodied needles and cutting needles.

Round-bodied needles

Round-bodied needles are designed to separate tissue fibres rather than cut them and are used either for soft tissue or in situations where easy splitting of tissue fibres is possible. After the passage of the needle, the tissue closes tightly round the suture material, thereby forming a leak-proof suture line, which is particularly vital in intestinal and cardiovascular surgery. Round-bodied needles are often used in obstetrics and gynaecology.

Blunt or taperpoint blunt needles have been proposed as a means of reducing glove puncture, especially in patients with blood borne viruses, and can be used in all layers of caesarean section except the skin. They are also used to suture tissues that are friable.

Cutting needles

A cutting needle is required where tough or dense tissue needs to be sutured. This needle has a triangular cross-section with the apex on the inside of the needle curvature and is useful for suturing tissues such as skin, tendon or scar tissue. Some needles combine the properties of a cutting needle and a round-bodied needle by limiting the sharp triangular cross-section to the tip, which then tapers out to merge smoothly into a round cross-section. This preserves the initial penetration of the cutting needle but also offers the minimised trauma of a round-bodied needle.

Needle size, shape and gauge

The choice of needle shape is frequently governed by the accessibility of the tissue to be sutured and the type of tissue. In a confined operative site, for example during vaginal surgery or deep in the pelvis, a greater curvature may be required with a smaller overall needle size. If access is open, such as an abdominal skin incision, then any needle type may be considered, even a straight needle. The wire gauge determines the strength of the needle; a relatively heavy wire gauge is used to suture uterine pedicles and fascial layers such as the rectus sheath.

Handling instruments

To achieve maximum potential from any surgical instrument, it will need to be handled correctly and carefully. The basic principles of all instrument handling include:

- safety

- economy of movement

- relaxed handling

- avoidance of awkward movements.

We shall demonstrate the handling of scalpels, scissors, dissecting forceps, haemostats and needle holders. Take every opportunity to practise correct handling, using the whole range of surgical instruments.

The scalpel

Handle scalpels with great care as the blades are very sharp. Practise attaching and detaching the blade using a needle holder. Never handle the blade directly.

For making a routine skin incision, hold the scalpel in a similar manner to a table knife, with your index finger guiding the blade. Keep the knife horizontal and draw the whole length of the sharp blade, not just the point, over the tissues (Figure 1.4a).

For finer work, the scalpel may be held like a pen. You can steady the hand by using the little finger as a fulcrum (Figure 1.4b).

Always pass the scalpel in a kidney dish. Never pass the scalpel point first across the table.

(a)

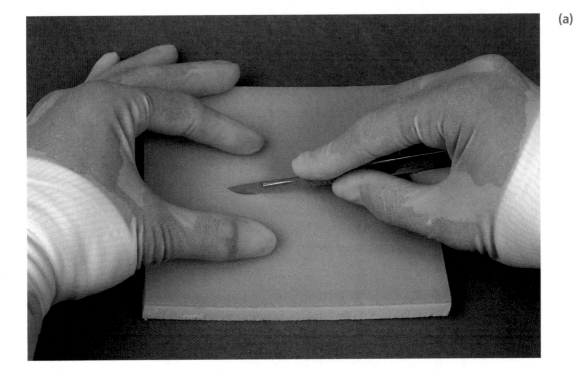

(b)

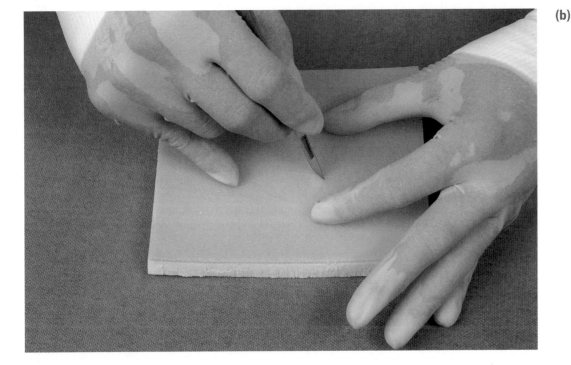

Figure 1.4 Holding the scalpel

Scissors

There are two basic types of scissors: curved for tissues that are soft and straight for sutures.

Insert the thumb and ring fingers into the rings (or bows) of the scissors so that just the distal phalanges are within the rings (Figure 1.5a). Any further advancement of the fingers will lead to clumsy handling and difficulty in extricating the fingers with ease.

(a)

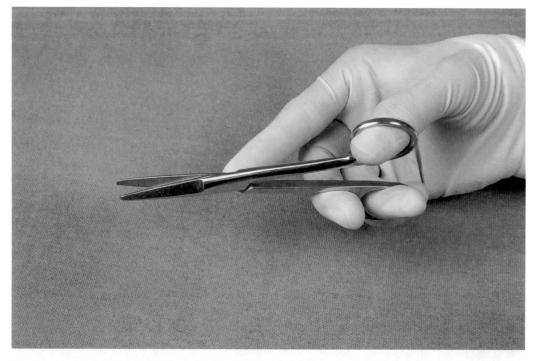

Use the index finger to steady the scissors by placing it over the joint.

When cutting tissues or sutures, especially at depth, it often helps to steady the scissors over the index finger of the other hand (Figure 1.5b).

(b)

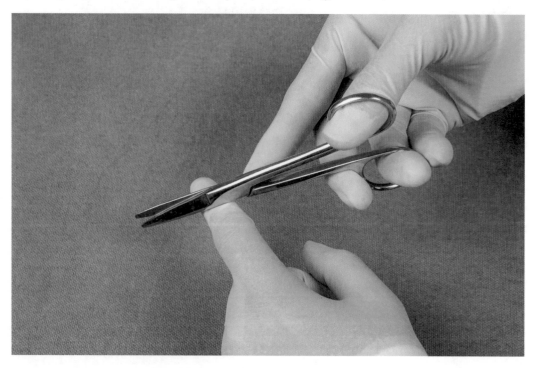

Figure 1.5
Holding scissors

Cut with the tips of the scissors for accuracy rather than using the crutch, which may run the risk of accidental damage to adjacent structures and will also diminish accuracy.

You should also practise cutting with the non-dominant hand and attempt to become surgically ambidextrous.

Dissecting forceps

Hold the forceps gently between thumb and fingers, the middle finger playing the pivotal role (Figure 1.6).

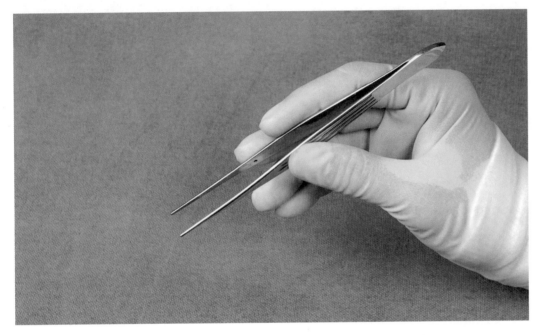

Figure 1.6
Holding dissecting forceps

Two main types of forceps are available: toothed for tougher tissue, such as fascia, and non-toothed (atraumatic) for delicate tissues such as bowel and vessels.

Never crush tissues with the forceps but use them to hold or manipulate tissues with great care and gentleness.

Artery forceps (haemostats)

Hold artery forceps in a similar manner to scissors.

Place on vessels using the tips of the jaws (the grip lessens towards the joint of the instrument).

Secure position using the ratchet lock.

Learn to release the artery forceps using either hand. For the right hand, hold the forceps as normally, then gently further compress the handles and separate them in a plane at right angles to the plane of action of the joint. Control the forceps during this manoeuvre to prevent them from springing open in an uncontrolled manner. For the left hand, hold the forceps with the thumb and index finger grasping the distal ring and the ring finger resting on the undersurface of the near ring (Figure 1.7) and gently compress the handles and separate them again at right angles to the plane of action, taking care to control the forceps as you do so.

Figure 1.7
Holding the artery
forceps

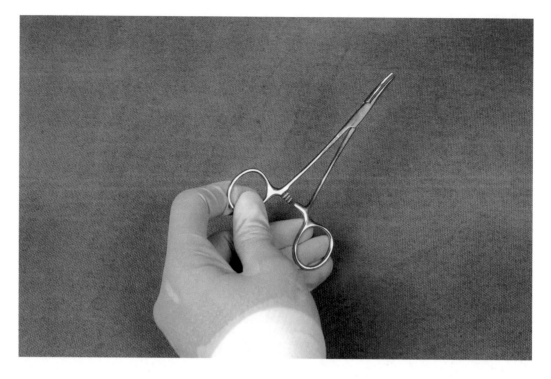

Needle holder

Grasp needle holders in a similar manner to scissors.

Hold the needle in the tip of the jaws about two-thirds of the way along its circumference, never at its very delicate point and never too near the swaged end.

Select the needle holder carefully. For delicate, fine suturing use a fine, short-handled needle holder and an appropriate needle. Suturing at depth requires a long-handled needle holder.

Most needle holders incorporate a ratchet lock but some, such as Gilles, do not. Practise using different forms of needle holder to decide which is most applicable for your use.

There is a wide variety of needle and suture materials available and their use will depend on the tissues being sutured.

PRACTICAL EXERCISE

Practise the correct handling of each of the instruments (scalpels, scissors, dissecting forceps, artery forceps and needle holders) as demonstrated.

Knot tying

Knot tying is one of the most fundamental techniques in surgery and is often performed poorly. Take time to perfect your knot-tying technique, as this will stand you in good stead for the rest of your career. Practise regularly with spare lengths of suture material.

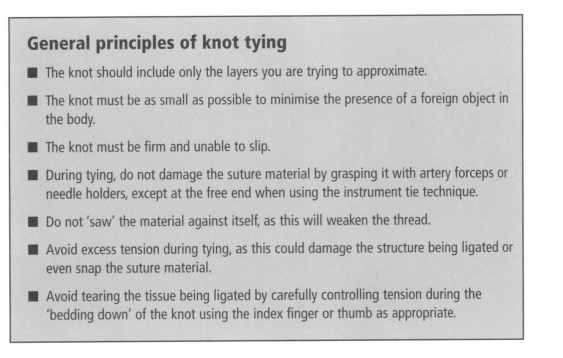

General principles of knot tying

- The knot should include only the layers you are trying to approximate.

- The knot must be as small as possible to minimise the presence of a foreign object in the body.

- The knot must be firm and unable to slip.

- During tying, do not damage the suture material by grasping it with artery forceps or needle holders, except at the free end when using the instrument tie technique.

- Do not 'saw' the material against itself, as this will weaken the thread.

- Avoid excess tension during tying, as this could damage the structure being ligated or even snap the suture material.

- Avoid tearing the tissue being ligated by carefully controlling tension during the 'bedding down' of the knot using the index finger or thumb as appropriate.

You will be taught and asked to demonstrate the following:

- the one-handed square knot

- an instrument tie square knot

- the surgeon's knot

- tying at depth

The square knot (reef knot)

The standard knot used in routine surgery is the square knot with a third throw for security. This can be tied using either the one-handed or two-handed method. The principles of the square knot are alternating ties of the 'index finger' knot and the 'middle finger' knot, with the hands crossing over for each throw. The single-handed technique will be the practised in the course (Figure 1.8a–h on page 18) but you should be familiar with tying the square knot with both a two-handed and single-handed approach.

The instrument tie

The instrument tie is useful when one or both ends of the suture material are short (Figure 1.9a–f on page 19).

The surgeon's knot

The surgeon's knot is sometimes used so that the initial throw remains secure before the second throw is made (Figure 1.10a–h on page 18). The disadvantage of the surgeon's knot is that it is less likely to tighten further with the second throw once an initial throw is made.

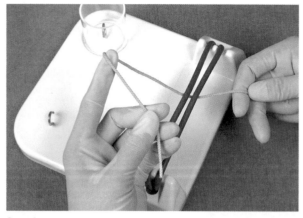

Step 1

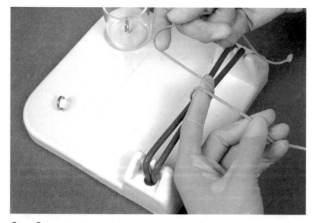

Step 2

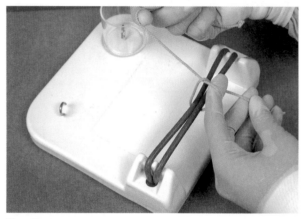

Step 3

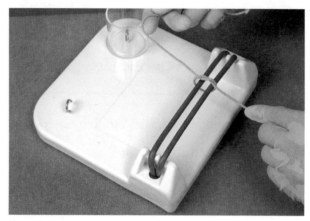

Step 4

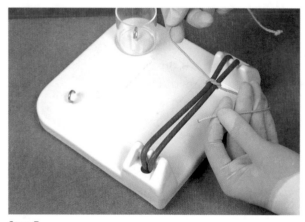

Step 5

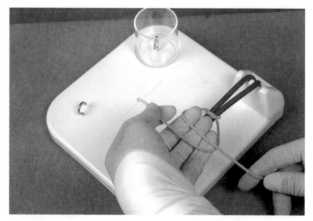

Step 6

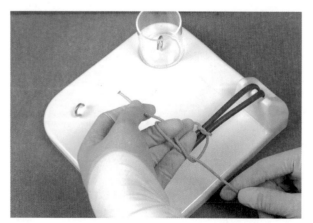

Step 7

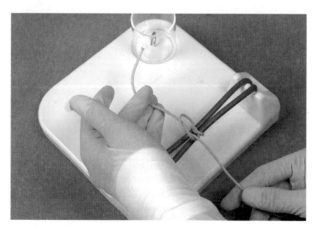

Step 8

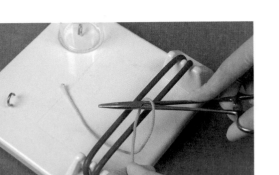

Step 1

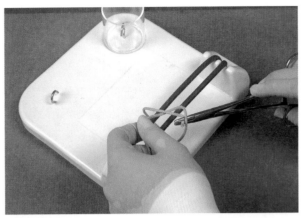

Step 2

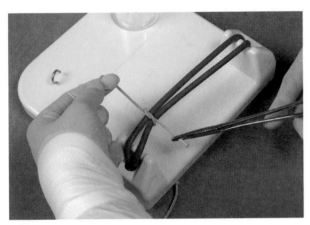

Step 3

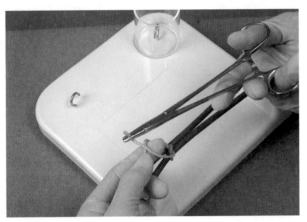

Step 4

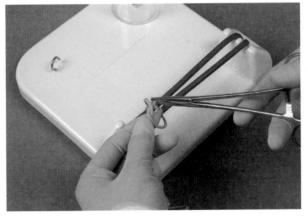

Step 5

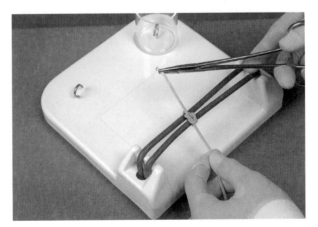

Step 6

Figure 1.8 (opposite)
The single-handed square knot

Figure 1.9 (above)
The instrument tie knot

Figure 1.10 (overleaf)
The surgeon's knot

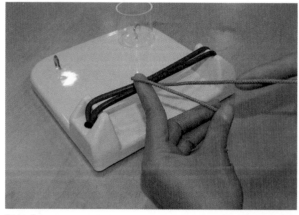

Step 1

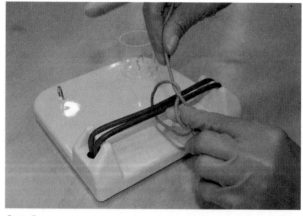

Step 2

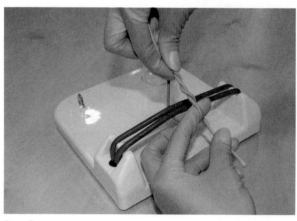

Step 3

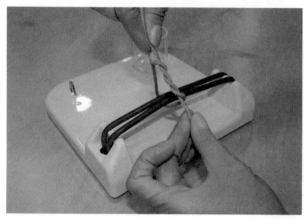

Step 4

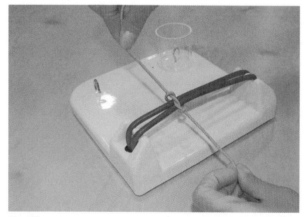

Step 5

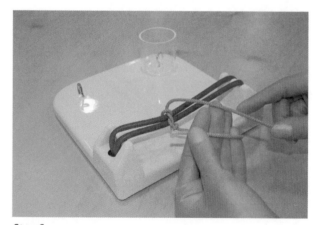

Step 6

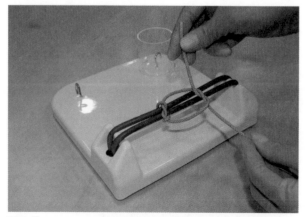

Step 7

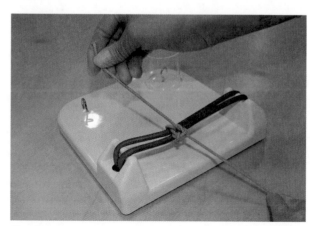

Step 8

Tying at depth

Tying deep in the pelvis or in the vagina may be difficult. The square knot must be 'snugged' down, as in all situations. The operator must also avoid upward pressure, which may tear or avulse the tissue (Figure 1.11a,b).

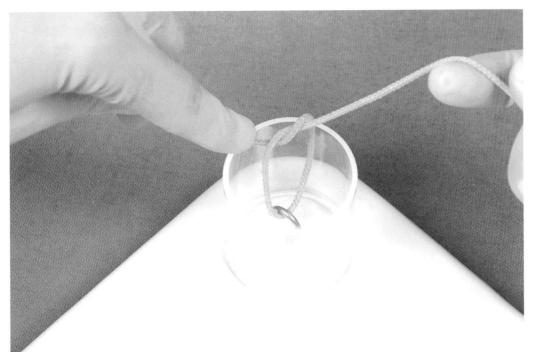

Figure 1.11
Tying at depth

(a)

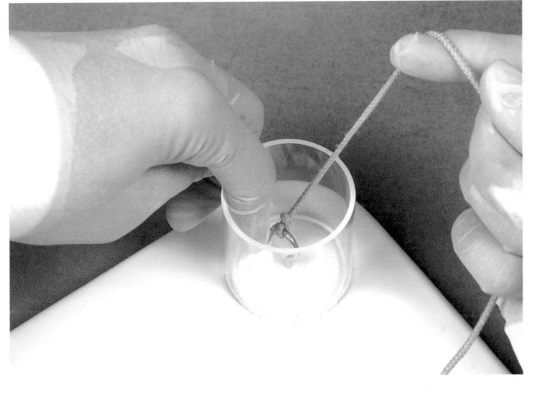

(b)

Principles of suturing

The basic principles of handling sutures are as follows:

■ Handle needles with instruments and not with your fingers.

■ Insert the needle at right angles to the tissue and gently advance through the tissue, along the curve of the needle, avoiding shearing forces.

■ As a rough rule of thumb, the distance from the edge of the wound should correspond to the thickness of the tissue and successive sutures should be placed at twice this distance apart, that is approximately double the depth of the tissue sutured (Figure 1.12).

Figure 1.12 Measuring the distance from the edge of the wound

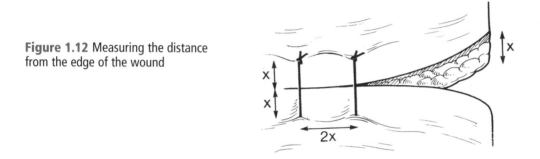

■ All sutures should be placed at right angles to the line of the wound at the same distance from the wound edge and the same distance apart for tension to be equal down the wound length. The only situation where this should not apply is when suturing fascia or aponeuroses, when the sutures should be placed at varying distances from the wound edge to prevent the fibres parting (Figures 1.13a,b)

Figure 1.13 Suturing fascia or aponeuroses

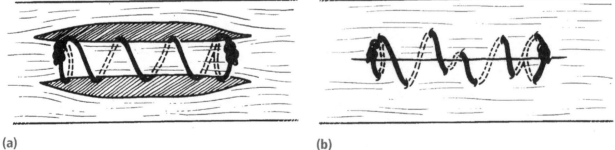

(a)   (b)

■ For longer wounds it is advisable that interrupted sutures are placed in the centre of the wound first, for accurate approximation of tissues.

■ No suture should be tied under too much tension. Too much tension results in oedema of the wound, which may delay healing.

■ In most cases, it is advisable to pick only one edge of the tissues at a time while suturing. If the edges lie in very close proximity and accuracy can be ensured then it is permissible to go through both edges at the same time.

■ A continuous 'locked' suture may be appropriate for uterine closure (caesarean section, myomectomy), as this spreads the suture tension and prevents the suture from tearing through tissue.

You will be taught and asked to demonstrate the following types of suturing:

■ interrupted sutures (including mattress and 'figure of eight')

■ continuous sutures (including locked and subcuticular)

■ The art of 'following'

Interrupted sutures

PRACTICAL EXERCISE

1. Place the suture carefully at right angles to the wound edges.

2. Tie a careful square knot and lay to one side of the wound.

3. Cut suture ends about 0.5 cm long to allow enough length for grasping when removing.

4. When removing sutures, cut flush with the tissue surface so that the exposed length of the suture, which is potentially infected, does not have to pass through the tissues below the skin (Figure 1.14b, 1.14c).

(a)

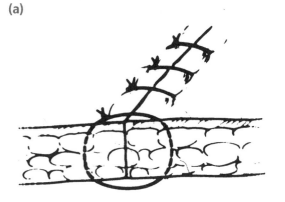

(b)

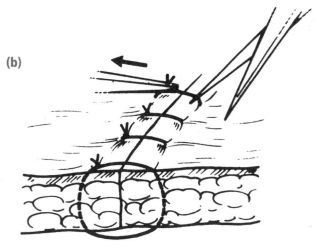

(c)

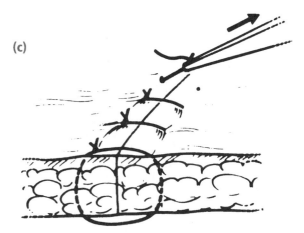

Figure 1.14 Interrupted sutures

Continuous sutures

Figure 1.15
Continuous locked
suture

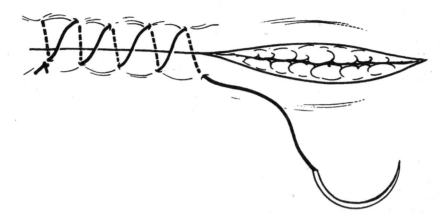

PRACTICAL EXERCISE

1. Place a single suture and tie a square knot but only cut the short end of the suture.

2. Continue to place sutures along the length of the wound. The assistant should maintain a steady tension while 'following' the suture.

3. Take care not to 'purse-string' the wound by too much tension.

4. Take care not to cause too much tension by using too little suture length.

5. Secure the suture at the end of the anastomosis by a further square knot.

6. You should also practise a continuous 'locked' suture; this is often used during uterine closure.

Mattress sutures

Mattress sutures may be either vertical (Figures 1.16a, 1.17a) or horizontal (Figures 1.16b, 1.17b). They may be useful for ensuring either eversion (Figure 1.16) or inversion (Figure 1.17) of a wound edge.

(a)   **(b)**

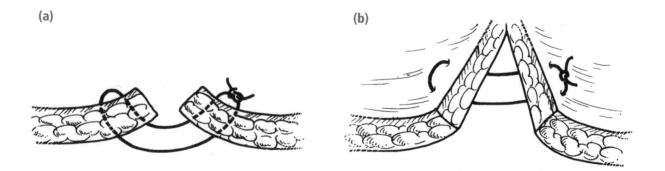

Figure 1.16 Eversion sutures (vertical and horizontal mattress)

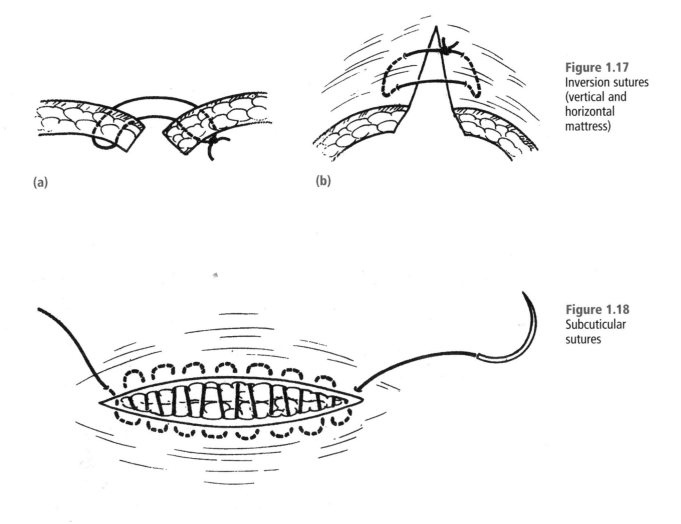

Figure 1.17
Inversion sutures
(vertical and
horizontal
mattress)

(a)　　　　　　　　　(b)

Figure 1.18
Subcuticular
sutures

Subcuticular sutures

Subcuticular sutures (Figure 1.18) may be used with absorbable or non-absorbable sutures. For non-absorbable sutures, the ends may be secured by means of beads, etc. For absorbable sutures the ends may be secured by means of buried knots. Small bites are taken of the subcuticular tissues on alternate sides of the wound and then pulled carefully together.

Anatomy of the anterior abdominal wall

Knowledge of the anatomy of the anterior abdominal wall is essential for both open and laparoscopic surgery. Consideration of the blood and nerve supply, muscles and underlying structures will limit complications during surgery and improve recovery.

Blood supply of the anterior abdominal wall

Superficial blood supply is derived from the femoral arteries. The deep blood supply is derived from the internal thoracic arteries from above and external iliac arteries from below.

PRACTICAL EXERCISE

Label the following vessels shown in Figure 1.19.

1.   Superficial epigastric vessels

2.   Inferior epigastric vessels

3.   Deep circumflex iliac vessel

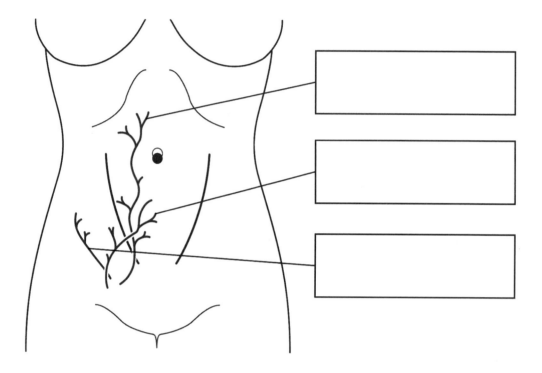

Figure 1.19
Label these
vessels

In view of the location of these vessels, where would you place the secondary (lateral) ports at laparoscopy?

The nerve supply

The nerve supply of the anterior abdominal wall arises from the thoracoabdominal, ilioinguinal and iliohypogastric nerves. Their branches cross superiorly to inferiorly as they pass in an arc and medially across the abdomen. Lower transverse incisions are often slightly curved to run between nerves and limit nerve damage, as well as creating a favourable cosmetic effect, as the incision runs along natural skin lines.

Abdominal wall muscles

The lateral muscles of the abdominal wall comprise of the external oblique, the internal oblique and the transversus abdominis muscles, which combine below the arcuate line to form the rectus sheath. The rectus abdominis muscle arises from the pubic symphysis and pubic crest and is attached to the costal cartilages. The pyramidalis muscle arises from the pubic symphysis and converges into the linea alba. The linea alba is a tough midline structure formed from fusion of the aponeuroses of all these structures.

PRACTICAL EXERCISE

Label the structures in Figure 1.20, which is a transverse section of the lower abdominal wall.

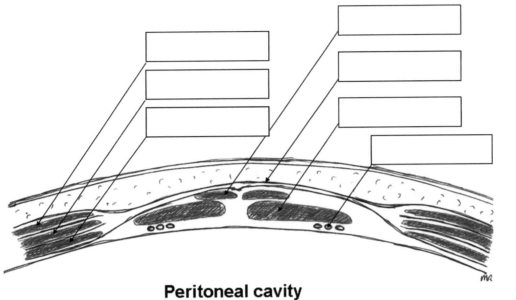

Peritoneal cavity

Figure 1.20
Label these structures

Surgical incisions into the abdomen

The main incisions used in gynaecology are the midline, suprapubic transverse (Pfannenstiel) and laparoscopic incisions (Figure 1.21).

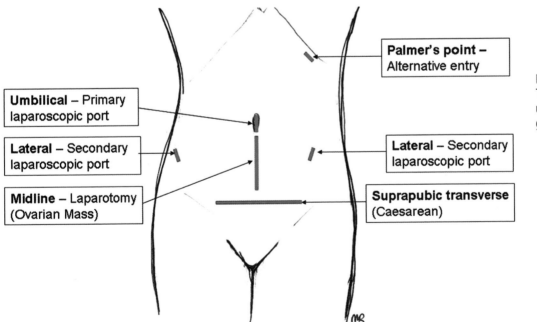

Palmer's point –
Alternative entry

Umbilical – Primary
laparoscopic port

Lateral – Secondary
laparoscopic port

Midline – Laparotomy
(Ovarian Mass)

Lateral – Secondary
laparoscopic port

Suprapubic transverse
(Caesarean)

Figure 1.21
The main incisions
used in
gynaecology

Midline incision

The midline incision incises through skin, subcuticular fat, the linea alba, transversalis fascia, extraperitoneal fat and peritoneum.

PRACTICAL EXERCISE

■ What are the indications for a midline incision?

■ What are its benefits?

■ What are the problems associated with it?

Suprapubic incision

The suprapubic transverse incision is an incision performed 2 cm above the pubic bone, extending beyond the lateral edges of the rectus abdominis. It is common to encounter superficial vessels within the subcutaneous fat of the lateral margins of the incision. The rectus sheath is then divided and reflected off the rectus abdominis muscle up to the level of the umbilicus and inferiorly well below the pyramidalis muscle. Perforating vessels are separated with diathermy and scissors. The muscles are divided in the midline and the peritoneal cavity is entered. The bladder should be avoided inferiorly. The approach used during caeasarean section often uses blunt finger dssection of most of the layers except the skin and the initial sheath incision (modified Cohen's incision). Variations in approach can be discussed with your supervisor or course facilitator.

PRACTICAL EXERCISE

■ What are the indications for a suprapubic transverse incision?

■ What are the benefits of this incision?

■ What are the problems associated with it?

Abdominal wall incisions for laparoscopic surgery

During laparoscopy, multiple small incisions are often made. Usually, the first incision is made at the umbilicus in the midline and subsequent incisions, lateral and suprapubic. The inferior epigastric vessels must be avoided during lateral port placement and these are best visualised directly through the laparoscope. In patients with previous abdominal surgery (in particular through a midline incision or for bowel surgery) bowel adhesions to the anterior abdominal wall can occur. A Palmer's point entry is through an incision in the upper abdomen on the left side, just below the lowest rib edge in the midclavicular line. This avoids the falciform ligament and bowel adhesions from previous surgery are uncommon. An alternative entry is an open (Hassan) subumbilical incision.

Practical exercises

Opening the abdomen

There are several layers of the abdominal wall including skin, subcutaneous fat, rectus sheath, muscle layer ond peritoneum. You will be provided with a simulator representing the abdominal wall with two layers of material, the innermost representing the peritoneum. They will be stretched over an inflated balloon, which represents loops of bowel within the peritoneal cavity. The aim of the exercise is to enter the peritoneal cavity without damaging the inflated balloon.

1. Make an incision in the simulated abdominal wall skin and subsequent layers (Figure 1.22).

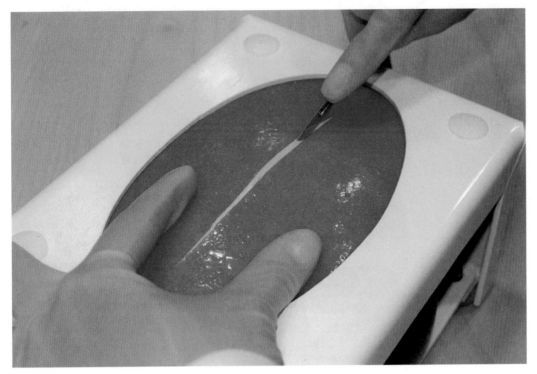

Figure 1.22
The initial incision

2. Expose the simulated peritoneum and lift up using artery forceps or tissue forceps (Figure 1.23).

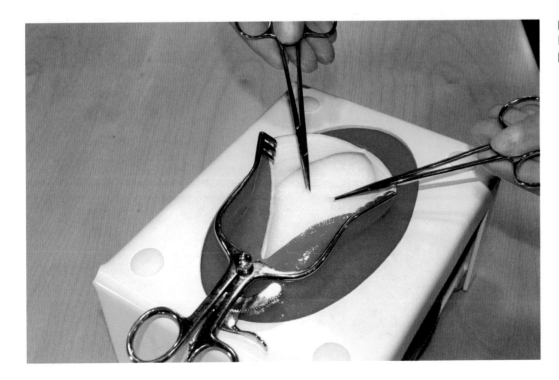

Figure 1.23
Exposing the peritoneum

3. Incise the peritoneum carefully ensuring no damage to the underlying balloon (Figure 1.24).

Figure 1.24
Incising the peritoneum

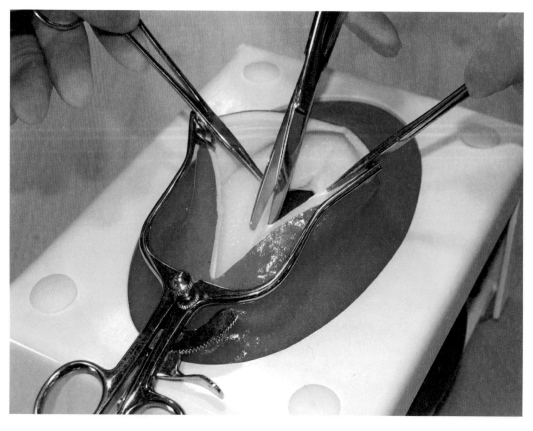

4. Enlarge the incision using scissors until the incision is adequate for the intended procedure (Figure 1.25).

Figure 1.25
Enlarging the incision

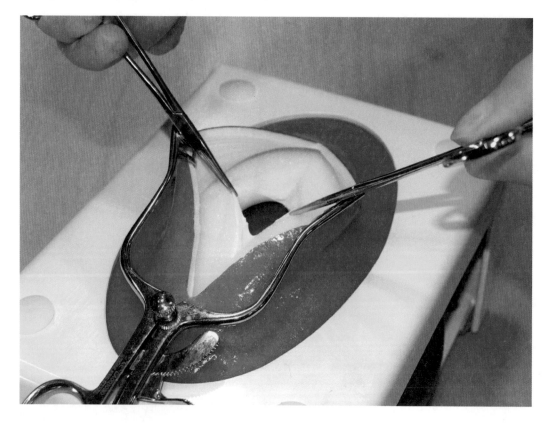

Closing the abdomen

The simulator already used in the above section for abdominal incision is used for this exercise. The two layers now represent the rectus sheath and the skin.

1. First insert a drain through all layers of the simulated abdominal wall. To do this, make a small skin incision to one side of the main incision. Pass an artery forceps bluntly through the incision to grasp the drain tubing without bursting the balloon and pull through the abdominal wall and fix the drain with a stitch on the skin.

2. Proceed to close the incision by inserting a number one (1–0) absorbable braided suture at one end of the incision, ligating the ends with the knot on the inside. Most surgeons would place at least one surgeon's knot. Some surgeons use a blunt needle for this procedure in order to minimise the risk of needle stick injuries.

3. Ensure that there is enough suture length to close the incision, which is normally four times the length of the wound. If the suture length is not adequate, a further suture can be inserted starting at the other end of the incision.

4. Close the entire wound meticulously, ensuring that no loop of bowel or tissue is caught up by the suture material (Figure 1.26).

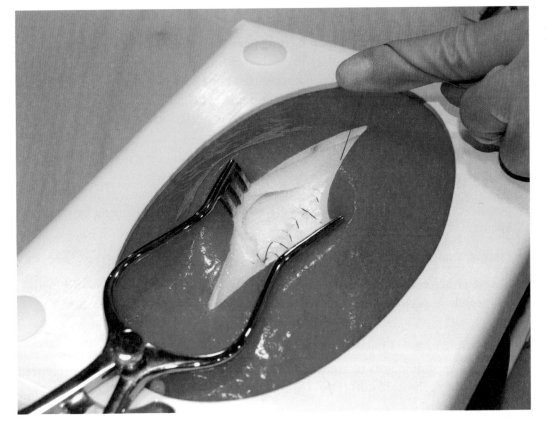

Figure 1.26
Closing the wound

5. Tie the suture material at the end of the closure.

6. The skin may then be closed, using an absorbable or non absorbable mono-filament subcuticular suture (Figure 1.27).

Figure 1.27
Closing the skin

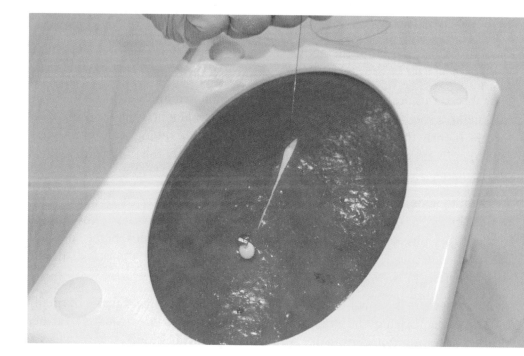

Haemostasis

There are several methods by which haemostasis can be secured. Two such methods will be demonstrated using simulated vessels in a model. If a vessel can be identified clearly and a pedicle created then haemostasis can be achieved by ligation (either with or without transfixing it). Otherwise a 'figure of eight' or 'box' stitch might be used where a vessel is difficult to identify (such as a uterine bleeding point during caesarean section).

PRACTICAL EXERCISE

Isolate a vessel in the model. Achieve a haemostatic suture by trying both of the following:

- Place a 'figure of eight' or 'box' suture (similar to horizontal mattress) across it.

- Isolate either end with a haemostat, divide the vessels between them and ligate the vessels in each haemostat with a three-throw reef knot.

OSATS

These exercises should now be considered in line with the RCOG Objective Structured Assessment of Technical Skills (OSATS) for Opening and Closing the Abdomen.

Full OSATS are available for download from the RCOG website: www.rcog.org.uk.

Module 2

Obstetric skills

Learning objectives

On completion of this module you will:

■ understand the anatomy of the pelvic floor and normal delivery

■ be able to demonstrate an efficient method of episiotomy repair

■ understand the principles of manual removal of the placenta

■ understand and demonstrate the principles of the instrumental vaginal delivery

■ be able to demonstrate fetal scalp blood sampling

■ be able to demonstrate a method for the management of shoulder dystocia

■ be able to manage major postpartum haemorrhage

■ understand the importance of surgical documentation.

Introduction

Many anatomical structures, such as the uterus and major blood vessels, are enlarged in pregnancy and the tissues are often soft, oedematous and easily bruised. This is particularly evident after a woman has given birth and can hinder the ready recognition of structures and tissue planes. As a consequence, surgery in pregnancy and in the postpartum period can be complicated by the rapid loss of a large volume of blood.

The trainee obstetric surgeon will become accustomed to operating in conditions of haemorrhage that would rarely be encountered in other surgical disciplines but this does not excuse poor operative technique. On the contrary, in order to function well in these difficult circumstances, the obstetrician must adopt a particularly careful and skilled approach to surgery. For example, it is important that you differentiate between bleeding inevitably associated with the conditions being managed and bleeding consequent upon poor technique. Tissues should be handled gently, meticulous haemostasis should be obtained at the earliest opportunity and divided structures should be reapproximated accurately and without tension.

In this module, you will learn about the anatomy of the pelvic floor and follow the normal vaginal birth of a singleton cephalic baby at full term. These topics should be revised before your attendance at the Basic Practical Skills course.

Three scenarios will be encountered on the obstetric day, as detailed at the beginning of the module. If you read the notes attached to each scenario before your training day you will gain most benefit from the experience.

Female pelvic anatomy

Detailed knowledge of female pelvic anatomy is essential to the obstetric and gynaecological surgeon. Without this knowledge, the risk of causing unintentional yet avoidable damage is considerably increased. In obstetric practice, for example, pelvic floor anatomy must be understood before the administration of a pudendal block, the application of a pair of forceps or the repair of an episiotomy can be mastered.

The pelvic floor

Figures 2.1 and 2.2 illustrate the pelvic floor, viewed from above and from below respectively. The pelvic floor may be likened to a funnel comprised of the levator ani muscles anteriorly and the coccygeus muscle posteriorly. Fascia covers these muscles and the term 'pelvic diaphragm' may be used when describing the combination of muscles and fascia together.

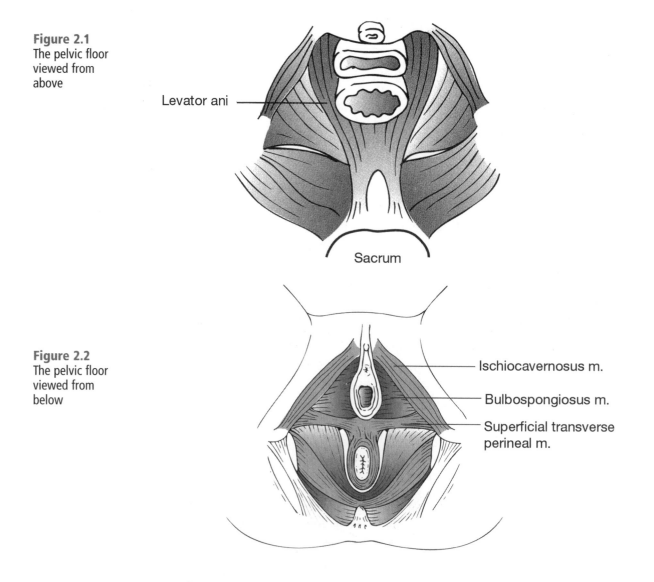

Figure 2.1
The pelvic floor viewed from above

Figure 2.2
The pelvic floor viewed from below

The anus lies at the apex of this funnel inferiorly while the vagina and urethra pass through the anterior aspect of the diaphragm. Passage through these apertures is controlled to a degree by muscular slings that act as sphincters, the most important of which is the external anal sphincter. This consists of three distinct muscular elements: a superficial ring encircling the anus, an intermediate component that slings around the front of the anus from behind and a deep component called puborectalis that slings behind the anus from the front. These must be meticulously and accurately realigned during perineal repair if they are damaged during childbirth.

The urogenital diaphragm

The urogenital diaphragm runs transversely below the funnel shaped pelvic diaphragm. The muscular component of the urogenital diaphragm comprises superficial and deep elements.

There are three superficial muscles:

- The bulbospongiosus (sphincter vaginae) surrounds the vaginal orifice. It interdigitates with the perineal body posteriorly and is attached to the corpora cavernosa of the clitoris anteriorly.

- The ischiocavernosus covers the unattached surface of the crus of the clitoris

- The superficial transverse perineal muscles run from the ischial ramus to the perineal body and complete the superficial element of the urogenital diaphragm.

There are two deep muscles:

- Deep transverse perineal muscles originate from the inner surface of the ischial ramus and insert into the perineal body.

- The sphincter urethrae surround the membranous urethra.

The perineal body

The perineal body, or central perineal tendon, is a fibromuscular mass that lies in front of the anal canal and behind the lower third of the vagina. Superficially it contains insertions of the superficial and deep transverse perineal muscles, the bulbospongiosus muscle and fibres of the external anal sphincter. Levator ani forms its superior aspect. It supports the vagina and anus as they exit the body and is prone to injury during childbirth.

The ischiorectal fossae

The right and left ischiorectal fossae (also known as Alcock's canals) are wedge-shaped spaces that occupy part of the lateral aspects of the perineum. The internal pudendal nerves and the pudendal blood vessels run through these fossae on each side of the pelvis. They are bound laterally by the obturator internus muscles, which cover the medial surfaces of the bony pelvis, and medially by the lateral surface of the levator ani muscles.

Figure 2.3
Mechanism of
labour

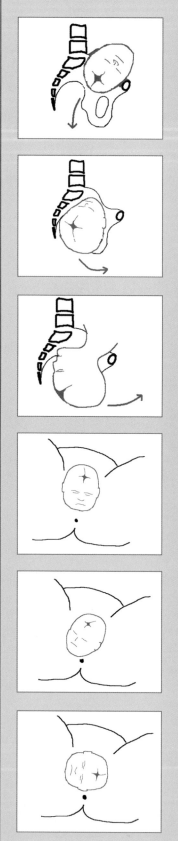

The head flexes as the uterus contracts.

The head descends and engages in the pelvis.

The leading part approaches the ischial spines.

The occiput starts to rotate anteriorly.

The occiput reaches the pelvic floor (levator ani).

Internal rotation continues to achieve an occipito anterior position.

The occiput clears the symphysis pubis.

The head extends to deliver.

The fetal head sits on the maternal perineum.

The fetal head realigns itself with the shoulders: **restitution**.

The shoulders come into contact with the pelvic floor and rotate so that the bisacromial diameter lies in a near anteroposterior orientation.

The head therefore continues to rotate: **external rotation**.

The pudendal nerve

Fibres of the pudendal nerve arise from S2, S3 and S4. The nerve passes between the piriformis and coccygeus muscles, curls around the ischial spine then re-enters the pelvis through the lesser sciatic foramen on each side of the pelvis. It thus comes to lie on the lateral wall of the ischiorectal fossa, medial to the pudendal artery. Obstetricians can use the close proximity of the pudendal nerve to the ischial spine to guide placement of a pudendal nerve block administered before instrumental vaginal delivery or episiotomy repair.

Spontaneous vaginal birth

It is estimated that the assistance of an obstetrician is required in less than 50% of all labours and births. The role of an obstetrician is to work harmoniously in a multidisciplinary team to minimise fetal, neonatal and maternal morbidity.

To do this effectively, we must first understand the mechanisms of spontaneous vaginal birth. As the fetal head descends through the pelvis, it undergoes the following passive changes in position and attitude (Figure 2.3).

Flexion

With full flexion, the posterior fontanelle is palpable near the centre of the cervix.

Internal rotation

The fetal head most commonly enters the pelvis in an occipitotransverse position. The occiput rotates anteriorly as it passes below the ischial spines, after coming into contact with levator ani.

Extension

Once the occiput passes beyond the pubic arch, the head begins to extend. The perineum is stretched as the head delivers.

Restitution

The head rotates approximately 45 degrees after delivery, realigning itself with the baby's shoulders.

External rotation

When the anterior shoulder reaches the pelvic floor, it rotates towards the symphysis pubis so that both shoulders come to lie near an anteroposterior plane. The fetal head follows this movement, thus returning to an occipitotransverse position.

Delivery of the shoulders

The anterior shoulder passes below the pubic symphysis to deliver, followed by the posterior shoulder then the rest of the baby.

Relative dimensions of the female pelvis and the fetal head

The average dimensions of the female pelvis are tabulated in Table 2.1. The widest diameter of the fetal head when it is well flexed is the biparietal diameter, measuring 10 cm on average. The rotation of the fetal head in the pelvis during labour results from its negotiation of a passage through the pelvis, under the influence of uterine contractions.

Professionals providing antenatal care to a pregnant woman should provide support and information about labour and should be ready to discuss with her all aspects of the birth process. Good antenatal care may maximise the chance of spontaneous vaginal delivery. In labour, the following measures may also be of benefit:

■ ensure that the bowel is not compacted with a large volume of faeces

■ ensure that the woman empties her bladder regularly

■ provide a form of pain relief that preserves some awareness of perineal pressure

■ maintain adequate uterine activity throughout labour

■ do not restrict the woman if she wants to adopt different positions when pushing.

Table 2.1
Dimensions of the mother's bony pelvis

Structure	Diameter (cm)
Pelvic brim	
Anteroposterior	11.5
Diagonal	12.0
Transverse	12.5
Mid-cavity (planes of greatest diameter)	
Anteroposterior	13.5
Diagonal	12.0
Transverse	12.5
Mid-cavity (planes of least diameter)	
Anteroposterior	11.5
Inter-ischial	11.0
Pelvic outlet	
Anteroposterior	9.5–12.0
Transverse	11.0

Scenario 1

Summary

Content

Phase 1: Ventouse delivery.
Phase 2: Manual removal of the placenta.
Phase 3: Episiotomy and its repair.

Reading material

Guidelines

RCOG Green-top Guideline Number 26: *Operative vaginal delivery.*
RCOG Green-top Guideline Number 23: *Methods and materials used in perineal repair.*
RCOG Green-top Guideline Number 29: *The management of third- and fourth-degree perineal tears.*

The latest versions of all RCOG Green-top guidelines are available to download from the RCOG website at **www.rcog.org.uk**

Record of progress

OSATS Operative Vaginal Delivery
OSATS Manual Removal of Placenta
OSATS Perineal Repair

Full OSATS are available for download from the RCOG website: **www.rcog.org.uk**

Phase 1

Case presentation

A 27-year-old primigravid woman with a singleton pregnancy and an uneventful antenatal history begins to experience regular painful uterine contractions near full term. The membranes rupture spontaneously shortly after her arrival at hospital. A midwife palpates the abdomen and finds that the fundal height is equivalent to dates. The presentation is cephalic with the fetal head 1/5 palpable per abdomen. On vaginal examination the cervix is found to be 4 cm dilated and the liquor is clear. Vertex presentation is confirmed and the head is thought to be well flexed, left occipitoanterior and at zero station.

An epidural is sited at the woman's request shortly after her examination and this provides adequate analgesia throughout the labour. There are no concerns about the fetal heart rate at any time.

The woman reaches full cervical dilatation 6 hours after arriving in hospital and 2 hours later active pushing is commenced. After a further 90 minutes, you are asked to assist as there seems to be little progress and the woman is exhausted.

You note that she is getting four good contractions every 10 minutes. On abdominal palpation the fundus is equivalent to dates and the fetal head cannot be felt per abdomen. On vaginal examination you find the cervix to be fully dilated and the liquor clear. The fetal head is well flexed with little caput or moulding, occipito-anterior and 2 cm below the ischial spines. The woman consents for ventouse delivery.

Ventouse delivery

The aim of instrumental delivery is identical whichever instrument is used: that is, to facilitate descent and delivery of the fetal head through the vagina. The most common indications are:

- fetal heart rate abnormalities
- low fetal scalp blood pH
- non-progressive labour in the second stage
- maternal exhaustion.

The main advantage of the ventouse over the forceps is that it is less commonly associated with maternal anal sphincter injury. The main disadvantage is that the ventouse has a higher failure rate in achieving vaginal birth than forceps.

Ventouse cups in current use include those made with metal (Figure 2.4), rigid plastic (Figure 2.5) and soft silicone rubber (Figure 2.6) materials. Cup widths vary between 50 mm and 60 mm in diameter. Suction tubing often arises from the centre of the cup but can also be from the perimeter, for use with occipitoposterior positions.

Figure 2.4
Metal ventouse cup

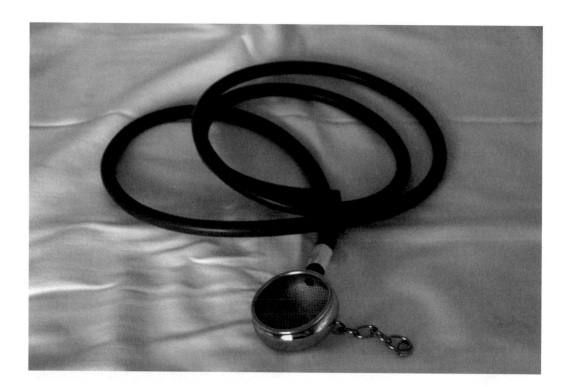

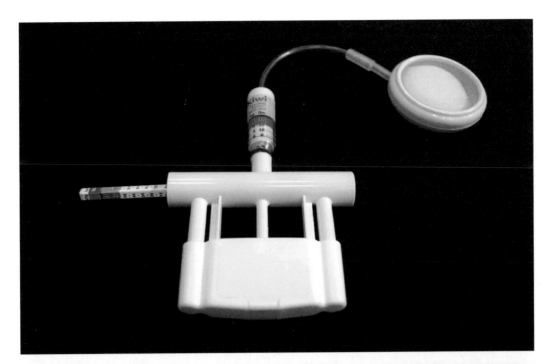

Figure 2.5
Rigid plastic
ventouse cup

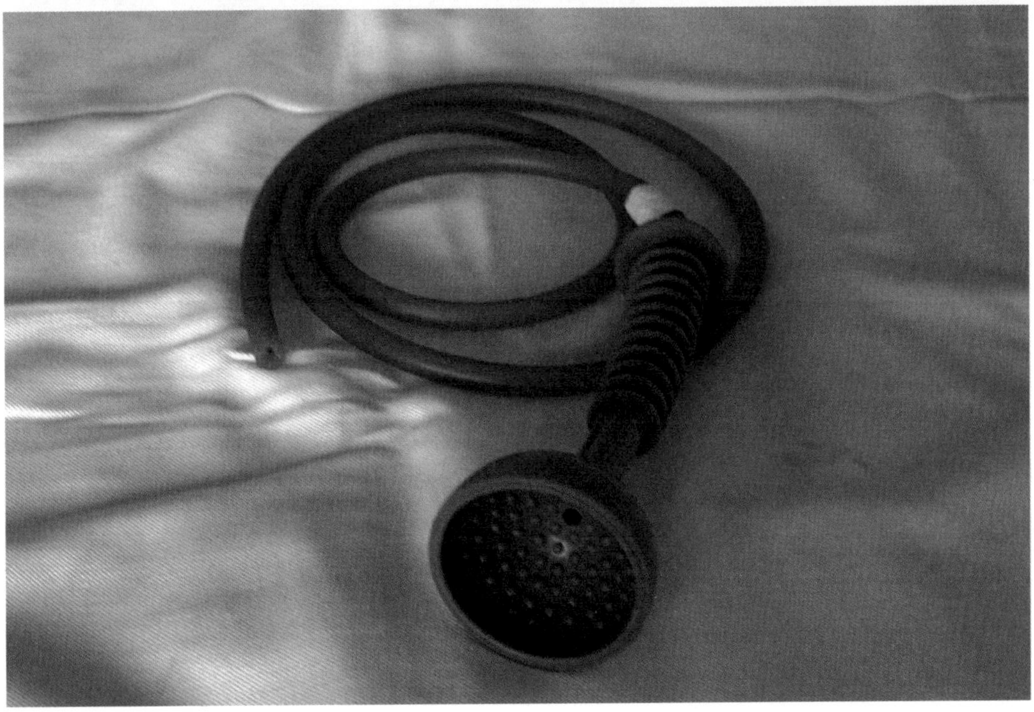

Figure 2.6
Soft silicone
rubber ventouse
cup

Ventouse delivery technique

Before applying the instrument:

■ Take consent. This means explaining the indication for the procedure, discussing its benefits and outlining its potential risks. Your discussion should be recorded on the partogram if not entered on to a formal consent form.

■ Ensure the woman has adequate analgesia (or local/regional anaesthesia).

■ Perform an abdominal examination. There should be no more than 1/5 of the fetal head palpable abdominally.

- Place the woman in lithotomy position. Clean the perineum and drape with sterile towels.

- Ensure that the bladder is empty.

- On vaginal examination, confirm that the cervix is fully dilated.

- Check the station of the presenting part. If this lies above the level of the ischial spines, instrumental delivery should not be attempted. The position of the fetal skull should also be defined. Note the presence and degree of caput in the soft tissues and moulding of the skull.

- Give your clinical impression of the capacity of the maternal pelvis but note that this cannot often be used to identify cephalopelvic disproportion.

For delivery:

- Check that the equipment can generate suction at the cup by testing it against the palm of your hand, using a negative pressure of $0.1 \, kg/cm^2$.

- Place the cup on the flexion point, 1 cm anterior to the posterior fontanelle in the midline, making sure that no maternal tissue is caught between the cup and the scalp.

- Activate the pump to provide a negative pressure of $0.2 \, kg/cm^2$ then recheck the cup position. Next, increase the pressure until $0.8 \, kg/cm^2$ is attained.

- Apply traction perpendicular to the plane of the cup. This will usually mean pulling the cup in a downwards direction initially then raising the handle of the cup as the head extends to deliver.

- Consider using an episiotomy when the perineum is well stretched. However, an episiotomy is not mandatory.

- Each pull should be synchronised with maternal contractions. Some descent should be apparent with each pull and delivery should be imminent or complete after three contractions. Delivery should take place within 20 minutes of the cup's application.

- If the cup avulses it can be reapplied up to two times but on each occasion check that you have not misdiagnosed the fetal position before reapplying the cup.

- After the procedure, carefully record all findings, indications for assisted delivery and the procedure itself in the notes.

PRACTICAL EXERCISE

Practise the ventouse technique on the mannequin.

Phase 2

Case presentation (continued)

As you deliver the baby, the midwife administers Syntometrine® (Alliance) for management of the third stage of labour. The placenta has not delivered 30 minutes later. There is little blood loss to be seen but you consent the woman for manual removal of the placenta and transfer her to theatre for the procedure.

PRACTICAL EXERCISE

- Describe physiological management of the third stage of labour.

- Describe active management of the third stage of labour.

- What steps might you take to deliver the unseparated placenta before transfer to theatre?

Whereas manual removal of the placenta rarely involves instrumentation of the uterine cavity, this is often required when a woman with secondary postpartum haemorrhage is thought to have retained products in utero. Good technique is vital if visceral injury is to be avoided.

Manual removal of placenta

When active management of the third stage of labour is being practised, up to 30 minutes should be allowed for placental separation unless significant bleeding is encountered. Ensure that the mother's bladder is empty, as a full bladder can often cause a retained placenta. After this time, manual removal is indicated.

- Take consent. This means explaining the indication for the procedure, discussing its benefits and outlining its potential risks. Your discussion should be recorded on a formal consent form.

- Ensure that adequate intravenous access is available and check the woman's full blood count. Group and save serum.

- Insert a bladder catheter as a full bladder can delay delivery of the placenta.

- Transfer to the operating theatre for an examination under anaesthesia.

- Check for the presence of a constriction band. Rarely, this may prevent delivery of the placenta. If a constriction band is present, the uterine tone could be relaxed with the aid of an inhalation anaesthetic.

- Otherwise, insert the dominant hand in the *main d'achoucher* position into the cavity. A plane between the placenta and uterine wall should be identified and the placenta separated and then removed. The other hand is placed on the abdomen over the uterine fundus and is used to prevent excessive movement of the uterus.

- If no plane of cleavage can be found, a morbidly adherent placenta may be present. Senior help should be sought as catastrophic haemorrhage can occur in such circumstances.

Phase 3

Case presentation (continued)

During the course of the ventouse delivery, you may have chosen to perform an episiotomy.

Episiotomy

There is no convincing evidence that the routine use of an episiotomy during spontaneous vaginal birth reduces the incidence of either anal sphincter injury or other significant perineal trauma, neither does it protect women from urinary dysfunction. In clinical practice, its use during ventouse delivery is variable. On the basis of expert opinion, however, episiotomy is recommended for protection of the anal sphincter during forceps delivery.

An episiotomy may be performed either in the midline from the vaginal orifice or mediolaterally. A right mediolateral episiotomy is the most commonly preferred option outside of the USA.

Adequate anaesthesia must be available to the woman. This will vary with clinical circumstances but may be achieved by:

- direct infiltration of the tissues with a local anaesthetic

- pudendal block

- regional blockade as part of another procedure.

Right mediolateral episiotomy technique

Seek verbal consent before performing an episiotomy.

Delay the episiotomy until the fetal head is stretching the maternal tissues. This will minimise blood loss from the operative site. Introduce your left hand into the vagina to guard the fetal tissues then make a right mediolateral incision using scissors during the course of a contraction.

The incision should arise from the fourchette. To avoid inadvertent injury to the dilated anal sphincter, it should be made at an angle of approximately 45 degrees to the midline. The size of the incision will vary with clinical circumstances but it is approximately 4 cm in length.

Episiotomy repair technique

The aim of episiotomy repair is to restore normal perineal anatomy without applying undue tension to the tissues. The repair must also achieve haemostasis. It should be undertaken as soon as possible after delivery to minimise blood loss and reactive tissue oedema.

Adequate anaesthesia is essential (see above).

The operative field must be adequately exposed and well lit. For this, excessive upper genital tract bleeding should be arrested before the closure is commenced. If a vaginal pack or tampon is used, a note of its insertion must be made by an attendant and its presence identified with a small clip on the attached tape. In some circumstances, the surgeon may need an assistant to hold back lax vaginal tissue with a right-angled retractor to ensure optimum view of the operative site.

- First, perform a combined vaginal and a rectal examination to define the extent of the injury. Gloves should be changed before continuing.

- Identify the apex of the incision and place the first suture 0.5 cm above this point.

- Next, repair the posterior vaginal wall with a continuous unlocked suture from the apex to the fourchette. The use of absorbable suture material such as polyglycolic acid (Vicryl®, Ethicon; Polysorb®, Covidien) is mandatory.

- Reconstitute the perineal body with continuous non-locking sutures, although interrupted sutures may be preferred for larger injuries.

- Close the perineal skin using a continuous subcuticular absorbable suture. Subcuticular sutures are associated with less pain than sutures penetrating the skin.

- Careful inspection should be undertaken to confirm adequate haemostasis.

- Combined vaginal and rectal examination must then be repeated to ensure adequacy of the repair and that bowel has not been included in the suture.

- All needles and swabs must be accounted for. The count and the procedure itself should be recorded in the notes.

If an episiotomy extends into the anal sphincter it is classified as a third-degree tear. If the anal mucosa is also breached, the injury is classified as a fourth-degree tear. Inexperienced obstetricians should not attempt to repair these injuries. Senior help should be sought.

If haemostasis is inadequate, a haematoma may form. This can extend into the pelvic side wall, causing considerable concealed loss of blood, delayed healing and pain. If a haematoma is identified, it should be assessed by a senior obstetrician: an actively evolving haematoma will require surgery for drainage and haemostasis while a stable lesion can occasionally be managed conservatively.

PRACTICAL EXERCISE

Complete an episiotomy repair, using the mannequin provided.

Scenario 2

Summary

Content
Phase 1: Pudendal block and forceps delivery.
Phase 2: Shoulder dystocia.
Phase 3: Postpartum haemorrhage.

Reading material

Guidelines
National Institute for Health and Clinical Excellence. *Intrapartum care: management and delivery of care to women in labour.* 2007.
www.nice.org.uk
RCOG Green-top Guideline Number 42: *Shoulder dystocia.*
RCOG Green-top Guideline Number 26: *Operative vaginal delivery.*
RCOG Good Practice Number 6. *The role of emergency and elective interventional radiology in postpartum haemorrhage.*

Record of progress
OSATS Operative Vaginal Delivery

Full OSATS are available for download from the RCOG website:
www.rcog.org.uk

Phase 1

Case presentation

A 22-year-old multiparous woman with a singleton pregnancy and an uneventful antenatal history is in established labour at full term. Fetal heart rate monitoring was initially by intermittent auscultation but a cardiotocograph was commenced when her midwife heard some decelerations after contractions.

You are asked to attend when the fetus suffers a bradycardia of unknown cause (Figure 2.7).

On examination, you find the fundal height to be equivalent to dates. The presentation is cephalic with the fetal head 0/5 palpable per abdomen. On vaginal examination, the cervix is fully dilated and the liquor is stained with meconium. Cephalic presentation is confirmed and the head feels well flexed, occipitoanterior and 2 cm below the ischial spines.

Entonox is currently being used for analgesia.

You roll the woman on to her left side and check her blood pressure, which is normal. After 3 minutes the baby's heart rate is not recovering so you decide that delivery of the baby would be wise. After discussion with the woman, you choose

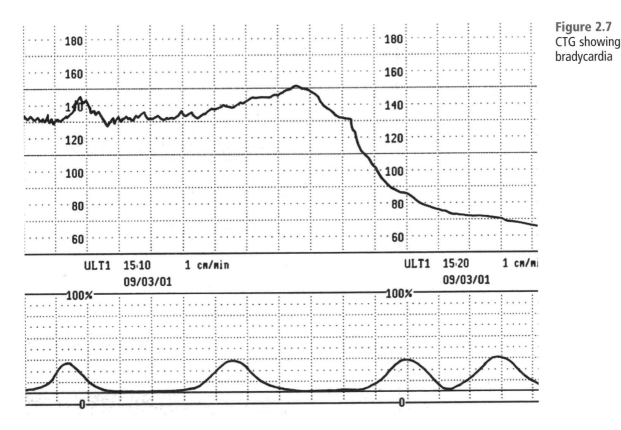

Figure 2.7
CTG showing
bradycardia

to use non-rotational forceps with a pudendal block for analgesia. The woman is encouraged to push while you set up your instrumental delivery trolley but this is not successful.

Pudendal block technique

To perform a pudendal block, the ischial spine must be located on one side of the pelvis by palpation during vaginal examination. A shielded needle is then introduced into the vagina between the maternal tissues and the operator's hand. Approximately 8 ml of 1% lidocaine is inserted into the tissue lateral to the ischial spine. The process is then repeated on the contralateral side. This will provide analgesia but the full effect may not be realised for up to 5 minutes.

You must withdraw the barrel of the syringe before injecting any local anaesthetic to ensure that the needle has not inadvertently punctured a blood vessel.

Non-rotational forceps technique

The traditional obstetric non-rotational forceps consists of two blades joined together at a non-sliding lock (Figure 2.8). Each blade has two curves: a cephalic curve, which allows the blade to fit around the fetal head, and a pelvic curve, which enables the forceps to be introduced into the curved passage of the pelvis. Compare this with the rotational forceps shown in Figure 2.9.

Before applying the instrument:

■ Take consent. This means explaining the indication for the procedure, discussing its benefits and outlining its potential risks. Your discussion should be recorded on the partogram if not entered on to a formal consent form.

Figure 2.8
Non-rotational
forceps blade

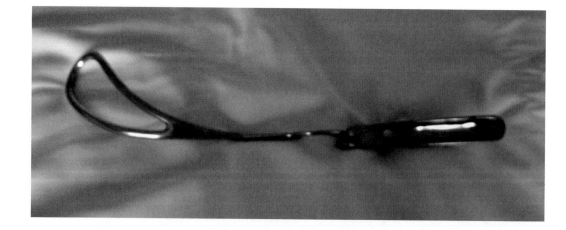

Figure 2.9
Rotational forceps
blade

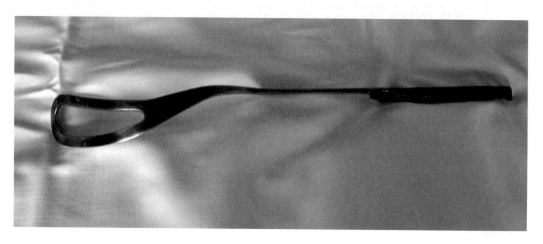

■ Ensure that the woman has adequate anaesthesia.

■ Perform an abdominal examination. There should be no more than 1/5 of the fetal head is palpable abdominally.

■ Place the woman in the lithotomy position. Clean the perineum and drape with sterile towels.

■ Ensure that the bladder is empty.

■ On vaginal examination, confirm that the cervix is fully dilated.

■ Check the station of the presenting part. If this lies above the level of the ischial spines, instrumental delivery should not be attempted. The position of the fetal skull should also be defined.

■ Note the presence and degree of caput in the soft tissues and moulding of the skull.

■ Give your clinical impression of the capacity of the maternal pelvis but note that this cannot often be used to identify cephalopelvic disproportion.

For delivery:

■ Check that your forceps blades are a matching pair by bringing them together and shadowing their application to the fetal head in front of the introitus.

■ Hold the left-hand forceps blade in your own left hand using a pencil grip, aligning the handle with the right inguinal ligament.

- Introduce your right hand into the vagina and feed the blade around the fetal head, guiding its application with your index finger and thumb.

- Repeat the procedure with the right-hand blade, mirroring these actions then locking the blades in the midline. The handles should be lying in a near-horizontal plane.

- Check that the sagittal suture can be felt in the midline and that no more than a fingertip can pass through each of the blades' fenestrations.

- With the next contraction, apply horizontal traction to the forceps with your right hand and vertical pressure with the left. This is Pajot's manoeuvre. It is designed to bring the fetal skull below the pubic arch.

- As the perineum stretches, perform a right mediolateral episiotomy. Lift the handles of the forceps gently as the head continues to descend, to reveal the face. Remove the blades when the chin comes into sight.

PRACTICAL EXERCISE

Practise non-rotational forceps on the mannequin provided.

Phase 2

Case presentation (continued)

After you have delivered the baby's head with your forceps, you try to deliver the shoulders with the next contraction using normal traction but cannot do so. Shoulder dystocia is diagnosed.

Shoulder dystocia

During the course of any vaginal delivery, the fetal shoulders usually deliver with a combination of maternal effort during a contraction and downward traction on the fetal head by the attending doctor or midwife. The force generated on the neck during this process will not usually be sufficient to cause damage to the nerve roots of the fetal brachial plexus.

Shoulder dystocia is the failure of shoulder delivery despite maternal effort and the use of normal traction on the head. The diagnosis can be inferred whenever additional maternal or fetal manoeuvres are needed to release the shoulders or whenever the accoucheur uses traction forces greater than is usual in his or her normal practice. The use of increased traction should be extremely rare.

Usually, the fetal shoulders deliver with a corkscrew action, rotating to the midline from a slightly oblique starting point. The cause of shoulder dystocia is impaction of the anterior shoulder behind the symphysis pubis. In severe cases, the posterior shoulder also becomes impacted on the sacral promontory. Disimpaction of the anterior shoulder or delivery of the posterior shoulder will almost always relieve the dystocia.

Shoulder dystocia is an obstetric emergency because it commonly causes compression of the umbilical cord. Good technique will reduce the duration of any hypoxaemia encountered while minimising the risk of fetal brachial plexus injury.

Risk factors for shoulder dystocia include:

■ previous history of shoulder dystocia

■ raised maternal body mass index

■ diabetes mellitus

■ fetal macrosomia

■ induction of labour

■ prolonged first stage of labour

■ prolonged second stage of labour

■ oxytocin augmentation of contractions

■ instrumental vaginal delivery.

Management of shoulder dystocia

The HELPERR mnemonic is often used as an memory aid in shoulder dystocia management.

At each stage of the process, try to deliver the baby for 30–60 seconds using normal traction.

Help	Call for obstetric, midwifery and paediatric support. Inform the anaesthetist.
Episiotomy	Evaluate for an episiotomy: this is to assist with later fetal manoeuvres. Moving the buttocks to the Edge of the bed may help delivery.
Legs	Place legs in McRoberts' position, hyperflexed at the hips and slightly adducted.
Pressure	Apply constant then rocking suprapubic pressure behind the anterior shoulder.
Enter	■ Place your finger behind the anterior shoulder and try to push this into the oblique. ■ Place your finger behind the posterior shoulder and try to push this into the oblique. ■ Try Woods' screw manoeuvre: continue the rotation a further 180 degrees. ■ A two-handed technique may be tried with any of these manoeuvres.
Remove	Remove the posterior arm: grasp the forearm and sweep it across the chest.
Roll	Roll the woman on to all fours then try to deliver the baby or repeat stages above.

This is a good starting point but a flexible approach should be adopted as you gain experience. For example, pushing the anterior shoulder into an oblique position and removing the posterior arm may be an equally effective intervention. Some authors argue that fetal manoeuvres are less likely to result in brachial plexus injury than maternal manoeuvres.

Figure 2.10 shows an algorithm for the management of shoulder dystocia, taken from RCOG Green-top Guideline No. 42.

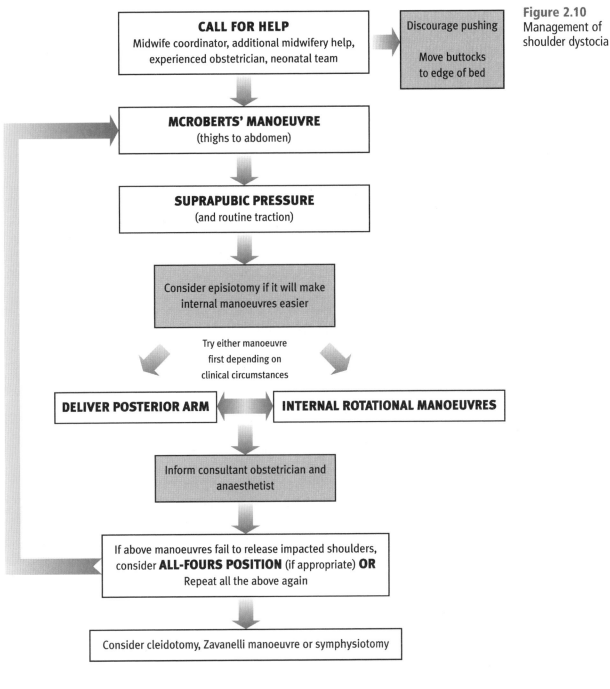

Figure 2.10
Management of shoulder dystocia

CALL FOR HELP
Midwife coordinator, additional midwifery help, experienced obstetrician, neonatal team

Discourage pushing

Move buttocks to edge of bed

MCROBERTS' MANOEUVRE
(thighs to abdomen)

SUPRAPUBIC PRESSURE
(and routine traction)

Consider episiotomy if it will make internal manoeuvres easier

Try either manoeuvre first depending on clinical circumstances

DELIVER POSTERIOR ARM   **INTERNAL ROTATIONAL MANOEUVRES**

Inform consultant obstetrician and anaesthetist

If above manoeuvres fail to release impacted shoulders, consider **ALL-FOURS POSITION** (if appropriate) **OR** Repeat all the above again

Consider cleidotomy, Zavanelli manoeuvre or symphysiotomy

Baby to be reviewed by neonatologist
DOCUMENT ON PRO FORMA AND COMPLETE CLINICAL INCIDENT REPORTING FORM

Other measures should be considered as a last resort, including cleidotomy, symphysiotomy and Zavanelli's manoeuvre. Only an experienced obstetrician should attempt these manoeuvres.

Minute by minute documentation is essential. This should be contemporaneous if possible, so an assistant is best placed to complete this record. You should also note whether the right or left shoulder was impacted and whether you used your normal traction for delivery or an increased traction force. The latter should be rare.

PRACTICAL EXERCISE

Practise your shoulder dystocia drill on the mannequin.

Figure 2.11
Major postpartum
haemorrhage drill

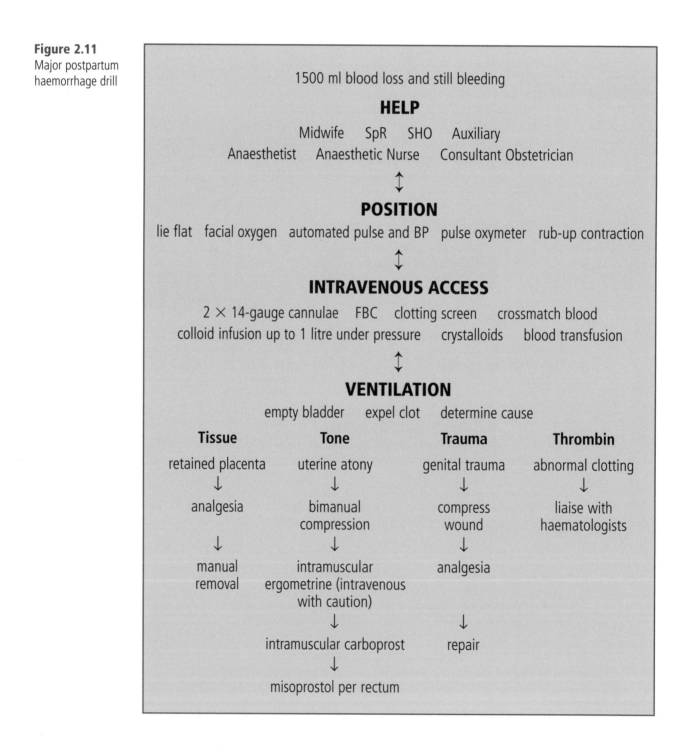

Phase 3

Case presentation (continued)

You release the baby's shoulders effectively by removal of the posterior arm and the baby is passed to the paediatrician for resuscitation. Syntometrine is given for the third stage of labour. Within 2 minutes of delivery, however, the woman experiences a rapid blood loss of approximately 1000 ml.

PRACTICAL EXERCISE

■ Define primary and secondary postpartum haemorrhage.

■ What are the causes of postpartum haemorrhage?

■ Your facilitator will now ask you to manage the case.

Postpartum haemorrhage

Primary postpartum haemorrhage (PPH) is the estimated loss of over 500 ml blood from the genital tract within 24 hours of delivery. It occurs after approximately one in ten births but is not always clinically significant.

Secondary PPH is the estimated loss of over 500 ml blood between 24 hours and 6 weeks after delivery. It occurs after approximately one in 100 births.

Major PPH is the loss of a large volume of blood after birth, often quoted as 1500 ml. It may occur within minutes but sometimes is not apparent for several hours. It is encountered in around one in 500 cases.

The causes of PPH may be remembered as **TTTT-I**:

Tone	Uterine atony.
Tissue	Retained placental tissue or membranes.
Trauma	Genital trauma, including damage to vulva, vagina, cervix or uterus.
Thrombin	Coagulopathy.
Infection	Secondary PPH is usually caused by or associated with ascending genital tract infection.

Major PPH remains one of the most common causes of maternal morbidity and mortality in the UK and elsewhere, so it requires prompt recognition and effective management:

■ be prepared to manage major PPH after any delivery

■ liaise with colleagues

■ use a locally agreed major PPH drill.

Management of major PPH

An example of a major PPH drill is given in Figure 2.11. This provides a guide to resuscitative measures that should be taken when managing major primary or secondary

PPH. In addition to the common initial steps, the specific causes of PPH should be assessed in each individual woman and action taken accordingly.

Tone

Try physical measures: expel clot from the uterus and vagina by rubbing up a contraction abdominally or bimanually compress the uterus.

Pharmacological options include ergometrine 500 micrograms intravenously immediately, carboprost 250 micrograms intramuscularly, repeated every 15–30 minutes up to a maximum of eight doses or misoprostol 800 micrograms rectally immediately. Intravenous ergometrine should be used with caution in hypertensive women. Once bleeding has been controlled and the circulating volume restored, an intravenous infusion of Syntocinon 20 iu in 500 ml physiological saline may be run in over 4 hours. There is no evidence for a reducing regimen.

If these interventions fail, transfer to theatre. You will generally start proceedings by examining the woman under general anaesthesia, looking for genital tract trauma or retained products. Further bimanual uterine compression can be attempted or tamponade tried, with a uterine pressure catheter (Rusch balloon/Bakri balloon) inflated with approximately 300–500 ml sterile water. Thereafter, laparotomy may be considered. Brace sutures (B-Lynch suture), internal iliac artery ligation and hysterectomy all have a roll to play in life-threatening PPH.

In some centres, embolisation of pelvic arterial vessels may be considered. This requires the services of an interventional radiologist and good access to specialised facilities.

Tissue

Try physical measures: manual removal of the placenta in the delivery room if the patient is unconscious or there is a dense regional block in place. If not, transfer to theatre for additional anaesthesia. If you have explored the uterine cavity manually, give an immediate dose of a broad-spectrum antibiotic such as co-amoxyclav 1.2 g intravenously.

If the cavity is empty and there is no evidence of other genital tract trauma, follow the atonic uterus guideline thereafter.

Trauma

Apply pressure over any easily identifiable bleeding point then suture it without delay. Transfer to theatre if the bleeding point is not easily identified or if the trauma is extensive.

If theatre transfer is needed, examine the anus, vulva, vagina and cervix under direct vision. Consider manually exploring the uterine cavity to exclude trauma or retained placental tissue. If these measures fail, follow the atonic uterus guideline.

Thrombin

Women with a preceding history of pre-eclampsia and antepartum haemorrhage are at particularly high risk of developing a coagulopathy. It may, however, complicate any case of PPH and should be presumed to have arisen in any major haemorrhage.

The diagnosis should be actively sought when bleeding continues despite the presence of an empty, well-contracted uterus and in the absence of genital trauma. Management with cryoprecipitate, fresh frozen plasma, platelets or recombinant factor VIIa will be determined on an individual basis after liaison with the on-call haematologist.

Blood transfusion

The decision to transfuse blood or other blood products, the volume of transfusion and the urgency required will be based upon several factors:

- estimated or measured blood loss
- continuing bleeding
- clinical condition
- response to colloid/crystalloid
- last-recorded haemoglobin.

Small women and women with pre-eclampsia are less tolerant of blood loss than others. A decision to use blood products should weigh potential benefits against potential complications including:

- transfusion reaction
- bacterial, viral or prion infection
- acute respiratory distress syndrome.

The attending obstetrician and the anaesthetist should discuss these factors and the outcome of this discussion should be recorded in the patient's notes. If the use of fresh frozen plasma, cryoprecipitate or platelets is being considered, the obstetrician or anaesthetist should liaise directly with an on-call haematologist:

- Transfusion of each unit of blood should begin within 30 minutes of retrieval from the fridge.
- Transfusion of each unit of blood should be complete within 2 hours of issue.
- Blood warmers should always be used.
- Unused blood should be returned to the blood bank promptly.

Recombinant factor VIIa

Recombinant factor VIIa (rVIIa) is occasionally useful in the treatment of women with major PPH. It should be considered when:

- life-threatening haemorrhage is continuing
- attempts to correct coagulopathy with other blood products have failed
- the fibrinogen count cannot be maintained over 1 g/litre
- the platelet count cannot be maintained over 20×10^9/litre
- internal iliac artery ligation or hysterectomy is being considered
- arterial embolisation is being considered
- the general management of the mother is otherwise optimal.

Note that when a woman who would refuse blood products has a major PPH, earlier recourse to rVIIa may be appropriate.

The use of rFVIIa should be approved by a senior haematologist. As many of these patients are seriously ill, early involvement of the duty intensive-care consultant is essential.

Scenario 3

Summary

Content
Phase 1: Intrapartum CTG interpretation
Phase 2: Fetal scalp blood sampling in labour
Phase 3: Caesarean section, including surgical documentation

Reading material
National Institute for Health and Clinical Excellence. *Intrapartum care: management and delivery of care to women in labour.* 2007.
National Institute for Health and Clinical Excellence. *Caesarean section.* 2004.
www.nice.org.uk
RCOG Clinical Governance Advice Number 6: *Obtaining valid consent.*
RCOG Consent Advice Number 7: *Caesarean section.*

Record of progress
OSATS Fetal Blood Sampling
OSATS Caesarean Delivery
Full OSATS are available for download from the RCOG website:
www.rcog.org.uk

Phase 1

Case presentation

A 31-year-old primigravid woman with a singleton pregnancy and an uneventful antenatal history is being induced because she is 14 days overdue. She receives one 3-mg vaginal tablet of prostaglandin E_2 because she has an unfavourable cervix. Over the next 6 hours she experiences mild backache.

Examination at this time reveals a fundal height equivalent to dates. Presentation is cephalic with the fetal head 1/5 palpable per abdomen. On vaginal examination, the cervix is 4 cm dilated and the membranes intact. Cephalic presentation is confirmed and the head lies at the level of the ischial spines. Amniotomy is performed then Syntocinon commenced to induce contractions. Thereafter, her contractions increase in frequency and duration. You suspect that she is in labour.

PRACTICAL EXERCISE

Look at CTG **A** below (Figure 2.12) and interpret it in the light of RCOG/NICE guidelines.

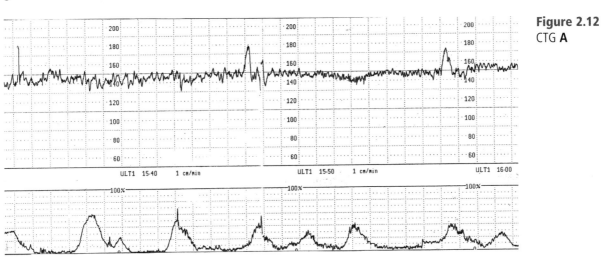

Figure 2.12
CTG **A**

The woman is examined an hour later by her midwife to assess progress. The cervix is now 5 cm dilated and the liquor heavily stained with meconium. The head feels deflexed, occipitoposterior and the presenting part remains at the level of the ischial spines.

PRACTICAL EXERCISE

Look at CTG **B** below (Figure 2.13) and interpret it in the light of RCOG/NICE guideline.

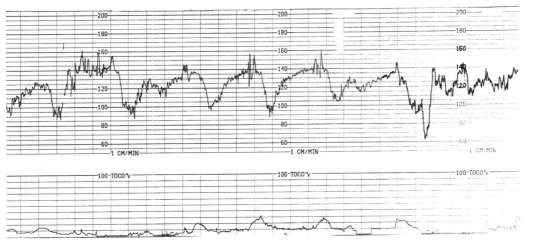

Figure 2.13
CTG **B**

CTG interpretation

The RCOG/NICE guideline suggests a scheme for the interpretation of a CTG for term babies in established labour. In this guideline, features of the CTG are defined as reassuring, non-reassuring or abnormal, while the overall impression of the CTG is defined as normal, suspicious or pathological. Tables 2.2 and 2.3 are taken from this guideline.

Table 2.2 Interpretation of features of the CTG

Feature	Baseline rate (beats/minute)	Variability (beats/minute)	Decelerations	Accelerations
Reassuring	110–160	Over 5	None	Present
Non-reassuring	100–109 161–180	Under 5 for 40–90 minutes	Early Typical variable	Absence is of unknown significance
Abnormal	Under 100 Over 180	Under 5 for over 90 minutes	Atypical variable Late	Absence is of unknown significance

Table 2.3 Overall impression and plan of action

Category	Definition	Action
Normal	Rate, variability and decelerations all reassuring	None
Suspicious	One non-reassuring feature	Conservative measures
Pathological	Two non-reassuring features or one abnormal feature	Fetal scalp blood sample or deliver the baby

Phase 2

Case presentation (continued)

You deduce that the CTG is pathological and decide to perform a fetal scalp blood sample.

PRACTICAL EXERCISE

Practise taking a fetal scalp blood sample using the simulator provided.

Analysis of duplicate samples provides the following results:

Sample 1   pH 7.14   Base excess –11.4 mmol/l
Sample 2   pH 7.16   Base excess –10.8 mmol/l

The clinical findings on abdominal and vaginal examination have not changed while the samples were being obtained and processed.

PRACTICAL EXERCISE

Discuss the results and make a plan of action.

Fetal scalp blood sampling technique

Fetal scalp blood sampling is useful when the fetal heart rate raises concerns. More specifically, sampling is required if the CTG is pathological but immediate delivery is not thought necessary. The cervix must be sufficiently dilated to allow the passage of an amnioscope and the fetal membranes must be absent.

Fetal blood sampling equipment varies from place to place and you should familiar-ise yourself with the equipment available to you before you start the procedure.

- Explain the procedure to the woman and obtain her verbal consent before proceeding.

- Ensure that the instruments are to hand and that the pH analyser is functioning.

- Place the woman either in a lithotomy position or in left lateral position with her right leg supported and abducted then drape the area around the perineum to provide a sterile field.

- Confirm the position and dilatation of the cervix by digital vaginal examination.

- Introduce the largest-diameter, lubricated amnioscope that the cervix can accommodate. Direct the amnioscope posteriorly then sweep it anteriorly to catch the anterior lip of the cervix.

- Remove the amnioscope's obturator and attach your light source. Ideally, the cervix should not be visible. Try to visualise the fetal scalp clearly.

- Clean the fetal scalp with a cottonwool ball dipped in sterile water then spray the scalp with ethyl chloride to produce a reactive hyperaemia.

- Apply a thin film of Vaseline® with a dental roll to increase surface tension on the fetal scalp; this encourages the formation of sizeable droplets of blood.

- Insert a guarded blade into the scalp to the full depth of the guard. Do not stroke the blade across the scalp as too large a lesion may be produced.

- Collect the blood droplet into your capillary tube. At least two samples should be obtained. The second may be taken while the first is being analysed by an assistant.

- Apply pressure to the fetal scalp with cotton wool at the end of the procedure if any bleeding is evident.

- Reposition the mother comfortably and explain the results to her together with your action plan.

Phase 3

Case presentation (continued)

You decide to deliver the baby by caesarean section.

PRACTICAL EXERCISE

- How will you convey the urgency of the procedure to your colleagues?
- What are the risks of the procedure?
- What should be recorded on your operation note?

Grade the urgency in caesarean section

The urgency of a caesarean should be determined by the attending obstetrician. This degree of urgency must be recorded clearly on the medical records and on the operation note. The form of anaesthesia will be determined by the anaesthetist after discussion with the attending obstetrician. The Obstetric Anaesthetists Association has devised the following grading scheme:

Grade 1 Immediate threat to the life of mother or fetus
Grade 2 Maternal or fetal compromise not immediately life-threatening
Grade 3 No maternal or fetal compromise but needs early delivery
Grade 4 Delivery time to suit mother and staff

Some of the conditions that may fall into each of these categories are listed in Table 2.4. The text gives one set of interpretations of this grading scheme but locally agreed guidelines are always recommended.

Table 2.4 Grading of urgency of conditions requiring caesarean section

Grade	Condition
1	Cord prolapse Uterine rupture pH ≤ 7.20 on fetal scalp blood sampling Antepartum haemorrhage with evidence of maternal or fetal compromise Pathological CTG when fetal blood sampling is inappropriate (e.g. profound prolonged bradycardia)
2	Failed instrumental delivery with no direct evidence of maternal or fetal compromise Antepartum haemorrhage with no direct evidence of maternal or fetal compromise
3	Malpresentation in labour with no evidence of fetal compromise Abnormal biophysical score with a normal CTG
4	All elective procedures

The time of the decision to perform a caesarean section should be recorded clearly in the medical records.

Consent

Think about consent as a process rather than as a signature on a form. This process involves:

■ informing the woman why a procedure is being proposed

■ giving her information about the possible complications of the procedure

■ providing her with clinically appropriate alternatives where they exist

■ making sure she understands the information given to her

■ giving her an opportunity to ask questions about the procedure

■ allowing her time to consider whether to undergo the procedure or not.

These principles apply for all surgical procedures in obstetrics and gynaecology.

For elective caesarean sections, this process is relatively easy to follow. The need for surgery may be discussed at leisure during the pregnancy, together with the alternative of an attempt at vaginal birth. Written information may be supplied to the woman about the risks and benefits involved. Written consent may be obtained by a suitably experienced clinician well in advance of surgery then simply confirmed by the surgical team before the operation itself.

The process is more difficult to follow when an emergency caesarean is being proposed; however, by definition, grade-2 and grade-3 caesareans are performed when there is no immediate threat to the life of the woman or her baby. In these cases, there should be sufficient time to discuss the risks and benefits of the procedure and to encourage the woman to ask questions. She may also benefit from being given time to reflect upon the proposed course of action before being asked to confirm her consent.

Obtaining consent for a grade-1 caesarean presents the obstetrician with a uniquely difficulty set of circumstances. Deterioration in the maternal or fetal condition may be expected as time passes. In this pressurised timeframe, you must ask a woman to consent to a procedure that will put her own health at risk yet may not be for her own direct benefit, as most grade-1 caesareans are performed for fetal rather than maternal concerns. Furthermore, the woman may be in pain or under the influence of analgesic drugs when asked to give her consent. Nevertheless, the principles above hold true. The indication for the procedure must always be conveyed to the woman and her consent confirmed, either in writing, verbally or by use of some physical means. In practice, the amount of time available for a full discussion of the risks and benefits of the procedure will vary with clinical circumstances, as will the time available to the woman for reflection.

Most women with low-risk pregnancies who are aiming for vaginal birth will achieve their goal. Some will not, however. To assist in the process of consent for grade-1, -2 or -3 caesareans, it is essential that all pregnant women receive information in the antenatal period about the indications for and potential risks of caesarean section. This can be achieved without posing a threat to normality in pregnancy and labour. It allows a woman time to reflect upon a procedure that she may eventually be offered and gives her time to have her questions answered.

Documentation of consent

The indication for any obstetric or gynaecological surgical procedure must always be discussed with the woman and clearly documented in her notes. In addition, any serious or frequently occurring potential complications must be discussed and documented, accepting that in an emergency some detail may be omitted.

Before caesarean section, the following potential complications might usefully be discussed and documented:

- intraoperative haemorrhage
- postpartum haemorrhage
- later return to theatre
- blood transfusion
- wound infection
- urinary tract infection
- venous thromboembolism
- bladder trauma
- trauma to the baby.

Women considering having a caesarean birth should be told that they are likely to have more abdominal pain but less perineal pain than women giving birth vaginally. It may also be more difficult to establish breastfeeding after caesarean section but, once established, birth by caesarean leads to no continuing disadvantage. Finally, the average length of hospital stay is longer after caesarean section than after vaginal birth.

The emphasis of this discussion will vary with the previous clinical history and present clinical circumstances.

Consent for anaesthesia should be obtained by an anaesthetist before the operation.

Operation note

The primary purpose of any operation note is to detail physical findings and surgical management but it may also be of great assistance in clinical management thereafter. It is worth remembering that an operation note is a legally admissible document.

These principles are correct for all surgical procedures whether a major pelvic procedure is being undertaken or a minor investigative procedure is taking place. The following points should be recorded, signed and dated on any surgical note:

- name of operation performed
- indication for the procedure
- form of anaesthetic
- surgeon (name and job title)
- surgical assistant (name and job title)   — Scrub nurse —
- anaesthetist (name and job title)
- incision site
- method of abdominal entry
- anatomical findings (all encountered structures, including abnormal findings)
- procedure   — Hand drawn Diagrams —   steps, difficulty, Hemostasis.
- closure
- plan for recovery
- plan for further treatment
- consensus of estimated blood loss   acc to Scrub Nurse & Anesthetist.
- swab count   } must be recorded
- needle count. } in Medical notes

Note that provision should be made to keep a record of all other people providing clinical care in an operating theatre during a procedure.

Free text may be preferable to describe the findings, procedure, closure of the wounds and plan of further action. In some cases, a pro forma may be of use as a memory aid. This most commonly applies to minor or repetitive procedures.

Blood loss is best estimated with the consensus of the scrub nurse and anaesthetist. Swab and needle counts must be recorded in the medical records but is often included with the scrub nurse's records.

Video or still pictures may be useful for the documentation of some abnormal findings, such as endometriosis diagnosed at laparoscopy. This may assist in the later assessment of disease response to medical treatment. Simple hand-drawn diagrams may also be used illustrate the findings and procedures undertaken.

Suggested reading

B-Lynch C, Coker A, Lawal AH, Abu J, Cowen MJ. The B-Lynch surgical technique for the control of massive postpartum haemorrhage: and alternative to hysterectomy? Five cases reported. *Br J Obstet Gynaecol* 1997;104:372–5.

Department of Health. Better blood transfusion: appropriate use of blood. *Health Service Circular* HSC 2002/009. London: DoH; 2002.

Drife J. Management of primary postpartum haemorrhage. *Br J Obstet Gynaecol* 1997;104:275–7.

Johanson R, Kumar M, Obhrai M, Young P. Management of massive postpartum haemorrhage: use of a hydrostatic balloon catheter to avoid laparotomy. *BJOG* 2001;108:420–2.

National Health Service Scotland. Better blood transfusion programme [www.betterblood.org.uk].

Sokolić V, Buković D, Fures R, Zadro M, Scurić I, Colak F, *et al.* Recombinant factor VIIa (rFVIIa) is effective at massive bleeding after caesarean section: a case report. *Coll Antropol* 2002;26 Suppl:155–7.

Module 3

Gynaecological procedures, hysteroscopy and laparoscopy

Learning objectives

On completion of this module you will:

- be able to undertake a gynaecological examination
- understand the principles of taking gynaecological swabs and cervical cytology specimens
- understand principles of intrauterine contraceptive device insertion
- understand principles of electrosurgery and methods of ensuring safe use
- be able to demonstrate basic hysteroscopy skills
- be able to demonstrate closed laparoscopic entry techniques
- have practiced laparoscopic manipulation skills.

Basic gynaecological examination and basic procedures

A gynaecological examination is an intimidating experience for most women. It should not be undertaken without prior training using a pelvic model. Having gained experience with the model, vaginal examination skills may be further developed (with consent), on the anaesthetised patient.

Always have a chaperone present when performing any kind of vaginal or pelvic examination. Ensure that the environment is as patient-friendly as possible by performing it in a warm, private and comfortable situation. Allow the patient to undress in privacy.

Most pelvic examinations are performed with the patient in the supine position on an ordinary flat clinic couch. Where procedures are anticipated, such as colposcopic examination, intrauterine contraceptive device (IUCD) insertion or hysteroscopy, it is preferable to use a gynaecology examination couch that facilitates examination in the lithotomy position or with legs supported. Transvaginal ultrasound is also often more informative using lithotomy.

Ensure that the appropriate equipment and instruments are available before approaching the patient; in particular, have a selection of different sizes of speculum to hand. For most nulliparous women, a small Cuscoe speculum is the optimal instrument; for most parous women you will need either a medium or large speculum to access the cervix adequately. When in doubt, it is occasionally worth performing a single-digit examination to assess introital capacity. This also allows the examiner to assess version and flexion of the uterus, which is important for speculum placement. In a woman with an anteverted uterus, the cervix is likely to be best visualised with the speculum in the posterior aspect of the vagina. In a woman with a retroverted uterus, the cervix is more likely to be placed anteriorly some centimetres distal to the vaginal vault. This is important information when deciding where to direct and when to open the Cuscoe speculum (Figure 3.1). If examination is difficult or painful, alternative patient positions (left lateral or lithotomy) or a different sized speculum should be considered.

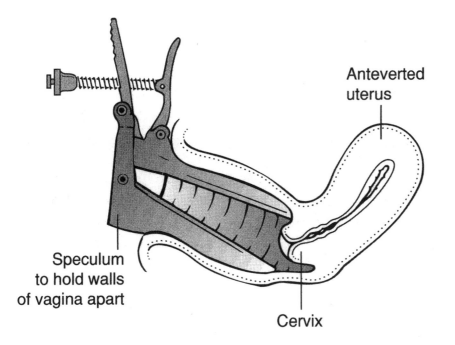

Anteverted uterus

Speculum to hold walls of vagina apart

Cervix

Figure 3.1
Inserting and opening the Cuscoe speculum

Speculae should have been adequately sterilised between patients. They should be warm and lightly lubricated (too little lubrication may incur unnecessary discomfort; too much may compromise the adequacy of cytological examination).

Inspection

The vulva and perineum should be inspected for scars, ulcers, lumps, discolouration, dermatological lesions of any kind, discharge or blood and for any signs of prolapse of the lower genital tract (see Figure 3.2 for a labelled diagram of the vulva). When inspecting the vulva, do so first with the labia untouched and secondly with them held apart. This allows you to inspect both the outer/lateral aspects of the labia and thereafter the introital area.

Figure 3.2
The vulva

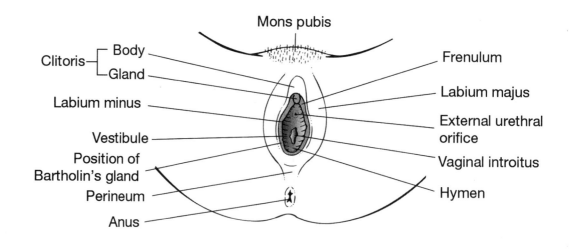

Before touching the vulva with either an examining finger or speculum it is usually wise to make physical contact with the patient elsewhere. Often, shaking hands will have achieved this with the patient at first introduction. The first physical contact between examiner and patient should not be the examiner's finger or speculum passing through the introitus.

Digital bimanual pelvic examination

The objective of the digital bimanual pelvic examination is to assess the pelvic organs and their normality. With the patient lying flat and with her legs apart, the examiner's left hand is used to separate the labia and allow the introduction of the index and middle finger of the examiner's right hand (this presuming the examiner is right handed).

Figure 3.3 shows the three different hand positions for a complete vaginal examination. In position 1, centrally, the consistency and position of the cervix is determined; in the nulliparous state the cervix is said to have the consistency of the tip of one's nose, whereas in the pregnant state it feels like one's lips. In position 2, anteriorly, the examiner can feel the size and position of the uterus in midline as well as the ovaries and adnexa in the lateral fornices. With the examiner's left hand pressing down transabdominally and the internal fingers pressing upwards and anterior to the cervix, towards the examiner's left hand, it is then usually possible to palpate the anteverted uterine body. In this way, the anatomical characteristics of the upper genital tract may be determined. The pouch of Douglas and both uterosacral ligaments are examined in position 3.

When documenting your examination findings, the size, version, consistency, shape, mobility and regularity of uterine outline should be included. A comment should always be made about the version of the uterus and whether any tenderness has been elicited. The normal parous uterus is the approximate shape and size of a small pear.

The ovaries may or may not be palpable in each adnexal area. Any adnexal masses should be documented and their size, shape, consistency and tenderness documented. The uterosacral ligaments should be sought and palpated for any masses, scarring irregularity or tenderness that might indicate disease in the pouch of Douglas, such as endometriosis.

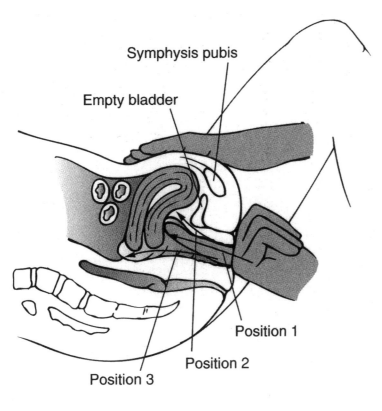

Symphysis pubis

Empty bladder

Position 1

Position 2

Position 3

Figure 3.3
The three positions for a complete vaginal examination

Speculum examination with Cuscoe speculum

The Cuscoe speculum allows visualisation of the vaginal walls and the cervix so that the cervix may be inspected, a cervical smear taken and other minor gynaecological procedures performed.

With the woman lying flat, the speculum should be inserted through the introitus in the transverse plane (that is, with the handles at nine o'clock). If inserted directly with the handle anteriorly, care should be taken to avoid contact with the urethral meatus and the clitoris. In this way, the blades of the speculum will enter the vagina in the anteroposterior plane (Figure 3.4a).

After insertion through the introitus and as the vaginal vault is approached, the handles of the speculum are rotated anteriorly from their lateral position until they are just off centre and thereby not in contact with the sensitive urethral meatus and clitoris. The blades of the speculum should now be opened under direct vision with an adequate light source whereby the cervix may be visualised (Figure 3.4b). The cervix comes into view when the speculum is opened (Figure 3.4c). The screw is tightened to retain the speculum in the correct position. This allows the examiner to free both hands. To remove the speculum, the handles are unscrewed and the blades withdrawn slowly. The vaginal walls help the closure of the blades but the handles should be held to prevent complete closure that can pinch the vaginal wall.

Speculum examination with Sims' speculum

In the outpatient setting, the Sims' speculum is usually used to assess the degree of genital tract prolapse. It is ideal for inspecting the anterior vaginal wall. With the woman in the left-lateral position and with her legs pulled slightly up so that she is

Figure 3.4
Inserting the
speculum

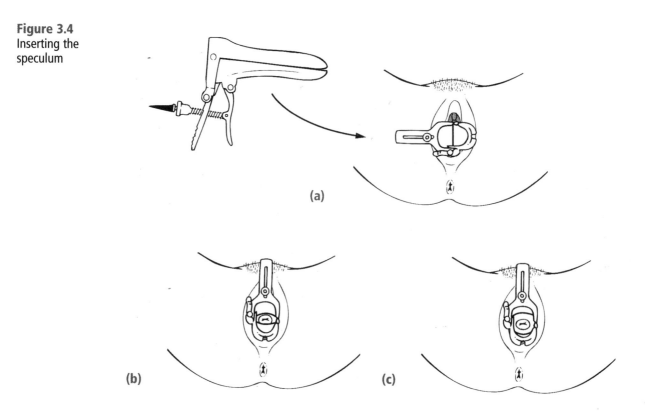

(a)

(b)   (c)

nearly in the fetal position, the curved speculum is inserted through the introitus and into the vagina. Once in the vagina, the speculum should be pressed down against the posterior wall thereby exposing the anterior wall (Figure 3.5). Reversing this manoeuvre allows inspection of the anterior wall. Alternatively, a sponge-holding forceps may be used to retract the anterior vaginal wall, while the Sims speculum is removed, allowing inspection of the posterior wall.

Taking a cervical cytology specimen (cervical smear)

Using a warm Cuscoe speculum and with the cervix fully visualised, a smear may be taken from the cervix. Do not routinely clean the cervix or take a swab before taking a cervical smear. Until recently, an Aylesbury spatula was used but liquid-based cytology (LBC) is increasingly available and a small brush is used in a similar manner to the old spatulae. The sampler should be inserted into the cervical os and rotated five times through 360 degrees using enough pressure throughout so that the sampler stays firmly applied to the epithelium of the transformation zone. The cytology brush is placed in a cytology transport medium or agitated to remove cells depending on the type of LBC method used. If using the old type of Aylesbury spatula, all the material is spread evenly over the whole of the non-frosted area of the slide on the **same** side as the patient's name and fixed immediately and generously. The final step is to ensure that the specimen and request form are labelled correctly and best done in the same room as the patient to verify the details.

Taking vaginal and endocervical swabs

Swabs should only be taken if clinically indicated or part of a screening programme. Unnecessary swabbing leads to detection of commensal organisms, such as haemolytic streptococcus and candida, which only require treatment if symptomatic or

Figure 3.5 Exposing the anterior wall

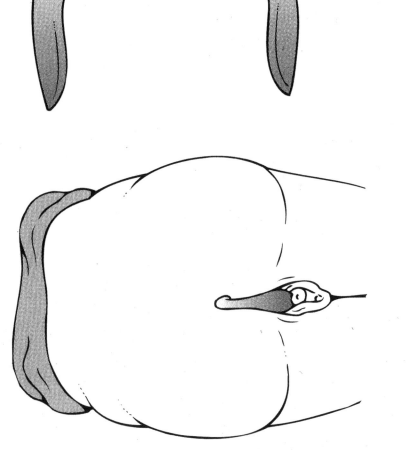

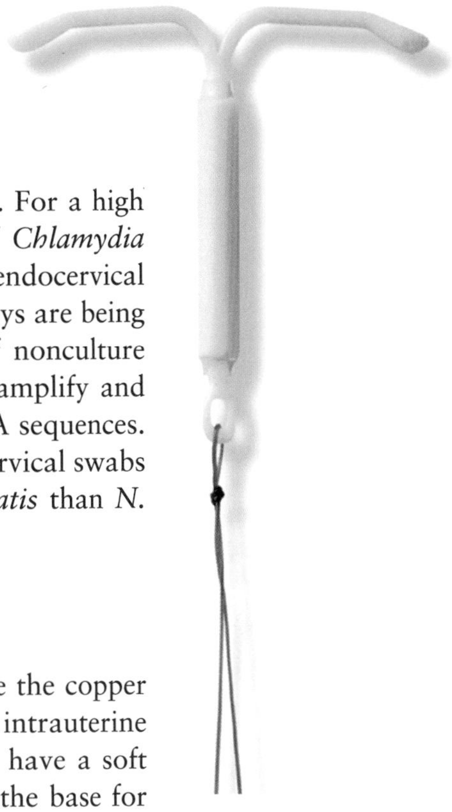

Figure 3.6
Intrauterine
contraceptive
device showing
thread for
retrieval

clinically indicated. The cervix is first visualised as documented above. For a high vaginal swab, a sample should be taken from the vaginal fornices. If *Chlamydia trachomatis*, *Neisseria gonorrhoeae* or endometritis are suspected, an endocervical swab is required. The old style of culture tests and enzyme immunoassays are being replaced by nucleic acid hybridisation tests. The latest generation of nonculture tests, called nucleic acid amplification tests, have been developed to amplify and detect *C. trachomatis*-specific or *N. gonorrhoeae*-specific DNA or RNA sequences. These tests are substantially more sensitive. Both can be used on endocervical swabs and urine specimens but are probably more reliable with *C. trachomatis* than *N. gonorrhoeae*.

Insertion of an intrauterine device

The most common intrauterine contraceptive devices (IUCDs) used are the copper intrauterine contraceptive device and the levonorgestrel-releasing intrauterine system used for contraception and menstrual disorders. Most devices have a soft plastic 'T' frame to hold the device in place and a thread attached to the base for later retrieval of the device (Figure 3.6). The risks at the time of IUCD insertion include infections and misplacement including uterine perforation. If pregnancy occurs then ectopic gestation should be considered.

Fitting of an IUCD is usually done with the woman awake. It can be painful and an intracervical local anaesthetic is often used. Some IUCDs are inserted under general anaesthesia, perhaps at the same time as other procedures. It is vital that the operator is fully trained to minimise pain, prevent introduction of infection or causing trauma.

A few hours before IUCD insertion it is often advised that the woman takes simple analgesics. After taking at least verbal consent for examination and IUD/IUS insertion, a bimanual examination (or transvaginal scan) is performed to identify the position and flexion of the uterus. The cervix is then visualised as discussed above. It is important that the cervix is cleaned under direct vision. If a local anaesthetic is used, a cervical block is achieved by injecting local anaesthetic just under the cervical skin at about 6 and 12 o'clock using a dental syringe. There is little evidence to suggest that a paracervical block reduces uterine sensation and may actually increase the risk of intravenous injection of anaesthetic agent.

After allowing a few moments for the anaesthetic to become effective, the cervix can be grasped using a tenaculum to steady the cervix and straighten the uterine axis for ease of IUCD insertion. The distance from the cervix to the uterine fundus is checked using a sound (Figure 3.7). This must be done gently to minimise pain and bearing in mind the axis and flexion of the uterus to prevent the creation of a false passage. (The IUCD will usually have an applicator, with which you should be familiar and should have practised using on a dummy uterus). The applicator containing the IUCD is gently inserted along the axis identified previously with the sound until the tip of the applicator reaches 5–10 mm from the fundus. The IUCD can then be released from the applicator and pushed the last few millimetres up to the fundus (Figure 3.8). The applicator device is removed and the threads cut so that they protrude through the cervix by about 2 cm. The speculum is removed and appropriate follow-up arrangements made.

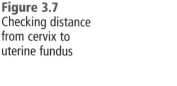

Figure 3.7
Checking distance from cervix to uterine fundus

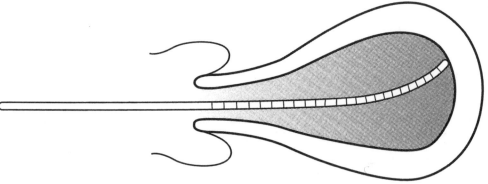

Spontaneous expulsion can occur, probably owing to associated trauma and infection, and placement should be checked after a first menstrual period and intermittently during its life.

Uterine evacuation

One of the most common procedures that trainees face is uterine evacuation for surgical management of miscarriage. The technique can be the same as for first-trimester termination of pregnancy.

Before undertaking a procedure it is essential that the operator has confirmation of 'non-viability' in line with local or nationally agreed Royal College of Radiologists/ RCOG guidelines (empty gestation sac with a mean diameter of greater than 20 mm or a fetal pole of 6 mm seen on transvaginal scan with no heart pulsation).

Uterine evacuation of retained products is usually performed under general anaesthesia in the UK. The principles of the procedure are as follows:

1. Prepare and drape the patient.

2. The bladder does not need to be emptied unless it is full, making it difficult to palpate uterus.

3. Undertake bimanual examination to determine position and size of uterus.

4. Visualise and grasp the cervix using a Sims' speculum and a tenaculum.

5. The uterus should **not** be 'sounded'.

6. If the cervix requires dilation, use graded dilators (it may already be open with incomplete miscarriage).

7. The 'rule of thumb' is that the gestational equivalent size of the uterus in weeks corresponds to the diameter in millimetres of the largest dilator used.

8. Retained products can be removed with a suction (Carmen) catheter with a diameter the same size as the largest dilator used. The catheter should be rotated within the uterine cavity to remove tissue, taking care not to perforate the uterine wall. Alternatively, a sponge-holding (Rampley's) forceps may be used to gently remove retained tissue in a piecemeal fashion.

9. Complete evacuation should be checked using a large uterine curette. The surfaces of the cavity should feel 'gritty' when curetted. Retained products would feel slimy.

10. Once the uterus is empty haemostasis is checked. If the uterus is 'boggy' or there is heavy bleeding, intravenous Syntocinon® (Alliance) 10 units should be given and, if necessary, bimanual compression of the uterus commenced until haemostasis is achieved.

11. The tenaculum and speculum are then removed. The operation is clearly documented, including total blood loss. Following miscarriage, products of conception are sent for histopathology assessment. After three consecutive miscarriages, some chorionic villi may be sent for cytogenetic testing.

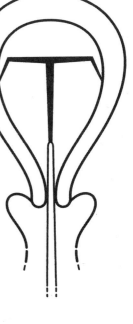

Figure 3.8
Releasing the IUCD

Suggested reading

Royal College of Obstetricians and Gynaecologists. *Gynaecological Examinations: Guidelines for Specialist Practice.* London: RCOG; 2002.

PRACTICAL EXERCISES

■ Gynaecological examination

■ Swab and smear taking

■ IUCD insertion

The use of electrical energy in surgery

Surgeons have used electrical energy for most of the last century. It is one of the most useful and adaptable surgical tools. It is also one of the cheapest modalities but it is also potentially dangerous. The dangers of electrosurgery are well recognised in conventional, open surgery but appear more marked when the energy is used laparoscopically, owing to the physical constraints of this approach.

It is essential that gynaecologists are formally trained in the use of electrical energy and that they understand the principles behind its safe use.

Whenever current passes through tissues, a heating effect occurs. The amount of heat produced depends upon the resistance of the tissue and the density of the current flow: the more current, the higher the tissue-heating effect. Tissues respond in a predictable manner to heat. An individual cell is irreversibly damaged when it is heated to a temperature above 45°C as the intracellular materials are denatured. Further heating will result in coagulation of proteins, which usually occurs at approximately 70°C and is visualised as a blanching of tissues. This is adequate for coagulation. Any further increase in temperature is likely to be detrimental. As the temperature approaches 100°C the intracellular water boils and the tissues can be seen bubbling and steam escapes as individual cells vaporise. When the tissue temperature rises further, residual tissue becomes carbonised and develops the characteristic 'charred' colour.

Key temperature points

45°C	Tissue death
70°C	Coagulation (blanching)
90°C	Desiccation
100°C	Vaporisation (bubbling)
200°C	Carbonisation (charring)

An understanding of the effects of heat upon tissue can be used to produce various useful surgical effects. If tissues are heated to a level just sufficient to drive off intracellular water the remaining proteins will become sticky. This is because the heat has produced a collagen chain reaction resulting in a fibrinous bonding of the denatured cells of the endothelium. If the walls of a blood vessel are firmly approximated during this process they will stick together. This is an effective method of sealing all but the very largest blood vessels and is widely used in both open and laparoscopic surgery.

Differing clinical effects can be produced either by changing the waveform of the current or more simply by changing the shape of the electrode (see page 76).

When a narrow band of high density current is focused on tissue it will completely vaporise the cells in which it comes into contact. This is most easily achieved when using a fine-pointed electrode held just above the tissue. This produces a cutting effect, which is the principle behind a cutting diathermy needle.

Coagulation will be produced when current is delivered through a broad electrode placed firmly in contact with the tissue. In such circumstances, heat is rapidly dissipated through a wide area, limiting the peak tissue temperature and so producing a diffuse coagulation effect.

It is important to understand that such cutting and coagulation effects can be produced by the same type of electrical energy on the same setting.

Monopolar diathermy

With monopolar diathermy, a small-sized active electrode produces heat at the operative site. The electricity is returned to the generator by passing through the patient and being dispersed by a return electrode placed on the patient's skin (Figure 3.9). This is usually the thigh in gynaecology, as the return electrode should be as close as possible to the primary electrode. To avoid a similar heating effect at the return electrode, it is essential that it is much larger than the primary electrode. With such a design, the current density will spread over a large area and become less concentrated so that the heating effect will be dissipated.

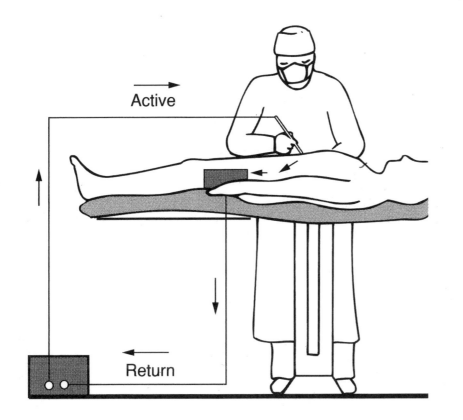

Figure 3.9
Monopolar diathermy

Bipolar diathermy

With bipolar diathermy, the primary and return electrodes are the two blades of the forceps, which are electrically insulated from each other (Figure 3.10). The current passes between the two electrodes and produces a relatively localised area of heating of tissue held between the blades of the device. No return electrode plate is required and there is less risk of burns at sites distant from the electrodes. This method involves intimate contact between the electrodes and tissue and the clinical effect is usually only of coagulation. This effect occurs despite the fact that modern bipolar generators deliver a continuous low-voltage, high-current 'cutting' wave form.

Figure 3.10
Biopolar
diathermy

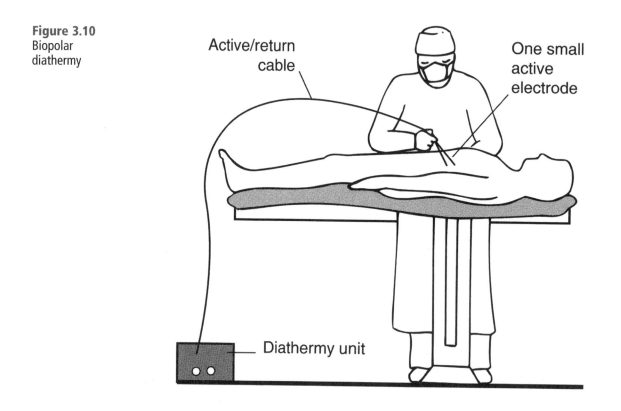

Active/return cable

One small active electrode

Diathermy unit

Good bipolar diathermy technique requires patience. The electrodes are usually fairly large and so the time required to heat tissue to the desired levels is significant. Attempts to speed up the process by turning up the power are likely to be counter productive. Higher energy levels will increase the local heat and char rather than desiccate the cells. Charred cells have a higher impedance, preventing further penetration of the heating effect. A satisfactory tissue desiccation should be associated with blanching and bubbling of tissue with slow release of steam. There should be no tissue charring. A good desiccation looks white and an unsatisfactory one is black.

Frequency of surgical current

It is well appreciated that connecting a human body to the electrical mains produces profound muscular stimulation. This Faraday effect may stimulate cardiac contractions sufficiently severe to cause cardiac arrest and death. This effect, however, only occurs when the frequency of the electrical cycle is relatively low. Mains current in the UK oscillates at 50 Hz (50 cycles/second). Fortunately for the surgeon, when electrical currents oscillate with a much higher frequency this neuromuscular stimulation effect is lost and current can pass through tissues without producing such effects. Electrosurgery, therefore, employs high-frequency currents with frequencies of up to 1,000,000 times that of the mains current. The frequency spectrum from household appliances to television can be seen in Figure 3.11. The frequencies used in electrosurgery are indicated.

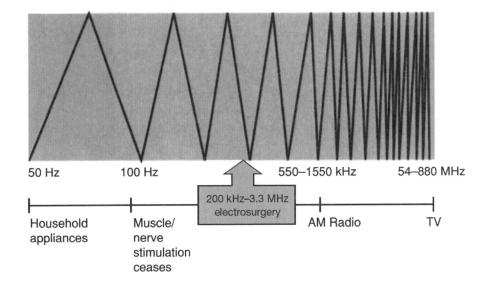

50 Hz   100 Hz   550–1550 kHz   54–880 MHz

200 kHz–3.3 MHz electrosurgery

Household appliances   Muscle/ nerve stimulation ceases   AM Radio   TV

Figure 3.11
Frequency spectrum of electricity in appliances

Waveform

In older electrosurgical generators, two types of electrosurgical energy were produced by two different mechanisms in the same machine. In modern electrosurgical generators, the form of the wave is altered electronically. We still use the terms 'cut' and 'coagulation' to describe these differing waveforms. A more accurate description for these would be unmodulated and modulated currents but the former terms appear to have become entrenched in our terminology.

With cutting current, the wave shape is a simple continuous sinusoidal form. When the power is switched on, the current flows continuously. The distance between the peaks and troughs of the wave form is fairly low, representing low peak voltage. Cutting current is therefore a high-current, low-voltage, continuous waveform. It is the fact that the current flows continuously which gives rise to the preferred term, unmodulated current. Cutting current is a confusing term because both cutting and coagulation effects can be achieved with this waveform, depending how the current is applied to tissue. If high-density current is applied a very short distance above tissue, it will jump the intervening space in the form of a spark, causing tissue vaporisation and a clinically useful cutting effect. If exactly the same current is applied directly to tissue with the electrode held firmly in contact with the underlying structures, a spark will not occur and instead the heat will be rapidly dissipated over a wide area producing a lower but more diffuse and gentler heating effect (Figure 3.12).

Coagulation current is more appropriately called modulated current because the sinusoidal waveform is non-continuous. As the total energy remains the same, interrupting the current increases the voltage. With coagulation or modulated current, pulses of current flow alternate with periods of no-flow and this provides a heating effect and thus coagulation of blood vessels. The longer the current is off, the higher the voltage in the periods of flow. Higher voltages result in a deeper heating and thus a greater coagulation effect.

Figure 3.12
The effect of electricity depending on surgical instrument electrode size

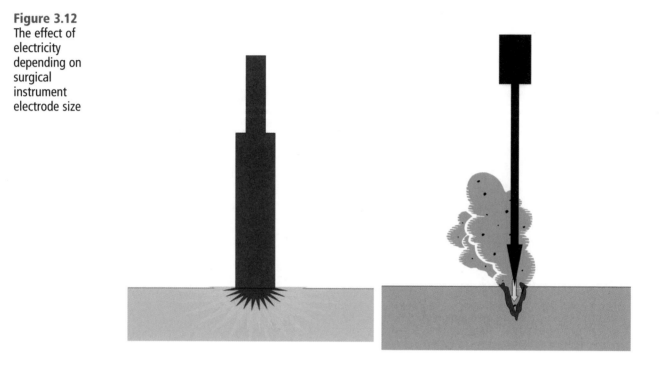

Some generators have three blends but these are being reduced or phased out in the newer generators. With blend 1, the current will flow for 50% of the time and off for 50%, in blend 2 it will flow for 40% and blend 3 for 25%. With each blend, the longer the time off the higher the voltage when the generator is activated. The extreme of this is when the 'fulguration' current is selected. In this position, the current is off for 94% of the time and the voltage can rise up to 5000 volts compared with 1000 volts for standard cutting current. Figure 3.13 shows the electrical wave forms of the pure cut, blends 1, 2 and 3, as well as the wave form of coagulation. Blends are classed as cutting waveforms and are activated using the yellow pedals, whereas the fulguration currents are classed as coagulation waveforms and activated by using blue pedals.

The blend modes result in greater time being required to produce a given cutting effect but should be selected when a greater haemostatic effect is required. The greater the haemostatic effect chosen the more associated collateral tissue damage, the greater the smoke produced and the greater the subsequent area of necrosis. A balance between precise tissue cutting and security of haemostasis must always be reached and it is preferable to reduce unwanted tissue destruction to the unavoidable minimum so that the risk of unwanted damage to important structures is also at a minimum.

The depth of tissue damage with electrosurgical heating is also limited by changes in the nature of the tissue being treated. As the intracellular water is driven out of cells, the impedance of the effected cells increases. Eventually, the impedance is so high that the current flow is insufficient to produce further heating and the surgical effect stops.

Risks of using electrosurgical energy

There are three sites of potential damage from the use of monopolar electrosurgery: the active electrode, the current diversion and the return electrode.

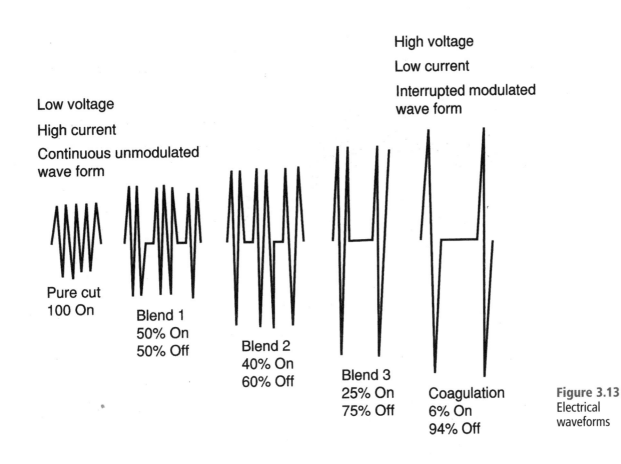

High voltage
Low current
Interrupted modulated wave form

Low voltage
High current
Continuous unmodulated wave form

Pure cut
100 On

Blend 1
50% On
50% Off

Blend 2
40% On
60% Off

Blend 3
25% On
75% Off

Coagulation
6% On
94% Off

Figure 3.13
Electrical waveforms

The active electrode is designed to heat tissue and cause tissue damage. Unintended burns may ensue if activated anywhere except the intended surgical site. It is important, therefore, to store such electrodes in an insulated holder at all times except when in use. They should not be left lying across the patient's abdomen nor held in the assistant's or nurse's hand.

Current diversion results because electrical energy will always find the path of least resistance to earth. If old earth-to-ground machines are used, the current may track down any metallic surface, such as a drip pole, leg support or even ECG electrode, if such structures are closer and lower in resistance than the return electrodes. If the size of these unintended return electrodes is not large enough to dissipate the resultant heat, skin burns will result. Engineers have solved this problem for us. Modern generators are isolated and this means that all energy leaving the generator is measured and all must return via the return electrode back to the generator. Any 'leakage' of electricity to earth will be detected and the machine will sound an alarm.

If the large-area return electrode is poorly applied or becomes partially detached from the patient, heating and burns at this site may occur. This problem has again been solved for us by the engineers. If a return electrode is divided into two halves and these halves are separately connected back to the generator, an interrogation current is sent across the two halves to measure the impedance between the two halves – split plate technology (Figure 3.14). If the plate partially detaches, the impedance rises and the machine alarm will be activated. Provided that modern single-use split electrodes are used this problem will not occur. Please ensure that you are using a modern, appropriate electrosurgical generator.

Figure 3.14
Split plate
technology

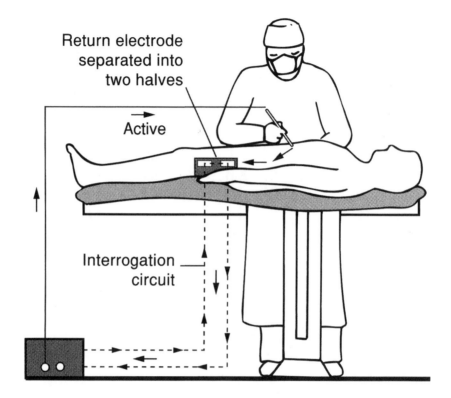

Safety check

✔ Always use isolated electrosurgical generator.

✔ Ensure no uninsulated metal comes into contact with the patient to provide alternative electrical pathways.

✔ Always use split-plate return electrode and check that it is properly applied.

✔ If the patient has a unilateral artificial hip joint, place the return electrode on opposite side.

✔ If the patient has bilateral artificial hips, place the return electrode on her back.

✔ If the patient has a cardiac pacemaker, avoid use of monopolar diathermy.

✔ Avoid placing return electrode over a scar or a bony prominence.

✔ Always place all electrodes in an insulated sheath when not in use.

Electrosurgery with laparoscopy

In addition to the factors listed above, there are two additional potential problems associated with the use of electricity in laparoscopic surgery:

■ the effect of introducing electricity through a cannula

■ the impact of the laparoscopic field of view.

Electrical energy, like all other surgical tools, must be introduced via tools inserted down cannulae. The structure of these cannulae can have a marked influence on the risk of electrosurgical damage.

Capacitative coupling

When two conductors are separated by an insulator, a capacitor is created. Thus, an insulated active electrode within a metal cannula forms a capacitor which can produce a 'capacitively coupled' electrical current that is transferred from the active electrode through the intact insulation into the metal cannula. Should the cannula come into contact with tissue, current is discharged which can damage that tissue. This phenomenon of capacitative coupling is well-known to electricians and engineers but seems a distant concept to most surgeons.

Problems arise if the coupled energy cannot escape and is stored in the cannula to take an alternative pathway of least resistance. Severe bowel burns have been produced in this manner. This unfortunate situation will occur when the metal cannula is insulated from the abdominal wall by a plastic thread mechanism (Figure 3.15c). Such mixed plastic and metal cannulae must be strictly avoided if used for electrosurgical work and only all-metal or all-plastic cannulae should be used (Figure 3.15a and b).

Insulation failure

The laparoscope permits only a partial view of the cavity. When used close up to the operative site only a very small proportion of the abdomen can be seen. Similarly, only the distal tips of most instruments, including electrical devices, are within the usual laparoscopic field of view. Most of the electrode will be out of view as it is activated (Figure 3.16). If there is a fault in the insulation on the shaft of the electrode, a severe bowel burn may occur without the operator being aware of it. Such burns are not usually recognised and can result in the most severe consequences. It is, therefore, important to perform visual and touch-test to confirm the integrity of the insulation, frequently, especially with reusable equipment.

Direct coupling

Direct contact between an active electrode and another conducting instrument can establish an unwanted and unnoticed current path. This is known as direct coupling and can occur in conventional as well as laparoscopic surgery. This can lead to serious visceral injuries outside the surgeon's field of view. The sparking and arcing are, however, more likely to be noticed with open surgery. In laparoscopy, the only sign is often that the diathermy does not appear to be working. Turning the power up in such circumstances can be disastrous.

Figure 3.15
Capacitative
coupling

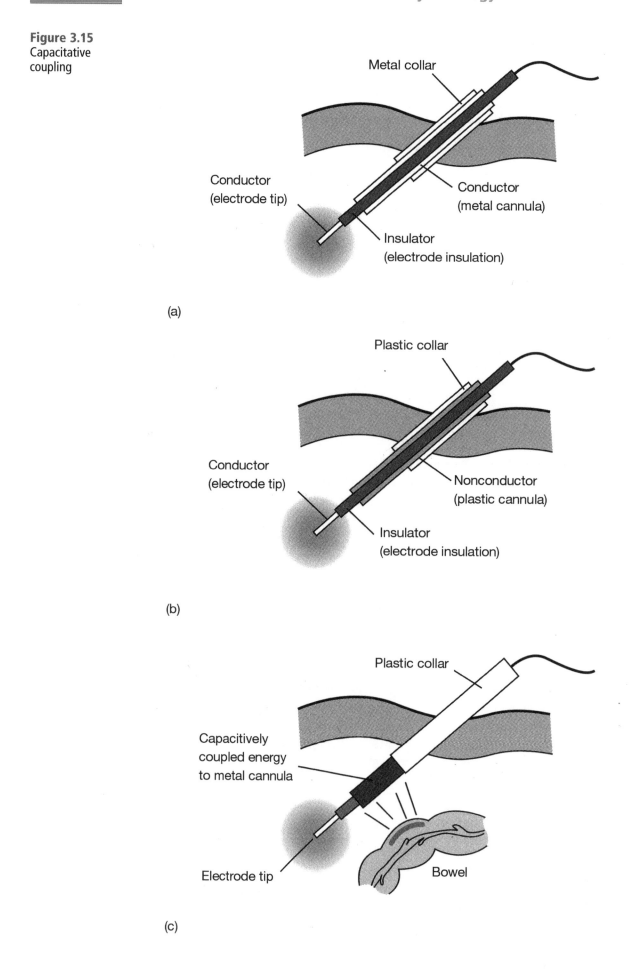

(a)

(b)

(c)

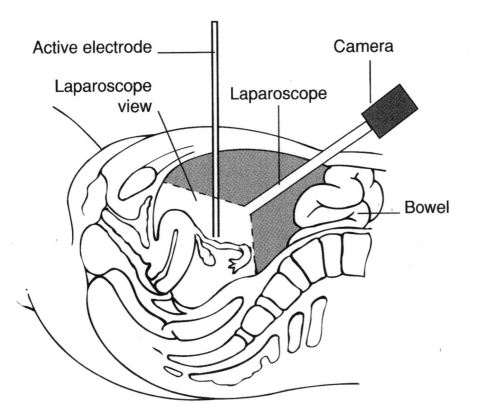

Active electrode

Laparoscope view

Camera

Laparoscope

Bowel

Figure 3.16
The active electrode is out of view

Safety rules

✔ Always use well-insulated electrodes and check the insulation before surgery if reusable.

✔ Only activate the electrode when its whole area which actively transmits current is in view.

✗ Do not activate the electrode when it is in contact with another conductor.

✔ Use all-metal or all-plastic trochars.

✔ Use low-voltage waveforms whenever possible.

✔ Use bipolar electrosurgery, wherever possible.

✔ Surgical smoke can be hazardous and should be sucked out carefully. A smoke evacuation system should be used to prevent theatre staff inhaling surgical smoke.

Electrosurgical energy is potentially dangerous but is a very useful surgical tool. Technological advances and improvements in understanding have made most po tential hazards avoidable. As with the use of any surgical tool, education and skill are required. This introduction to the principles of safe electrosurgery should help you to acquire the necessary information and skills.

Basic laparoscopy and hysteroscopy

Endoscopic surgery provides benefits for patients, with reduced postoperative pain and a more rapid return to normal life. For surgeons, the magnified view of pelvic structures is a great help. It is important that you understand how all the endoscopic equipment is used in the operating theatre. This will help you to operate safely and to identify technical problems.

Consenting patients for laparoscopic surgery and hysteroscopic surgery requires knowledge of complications that can happen with all endoscopic procedures, as well as the specific complications of each operation undertaken.

Early discharge from hospital is planned and achieved for patients who have had endoscopic surgery but it is important that patients are aware of what to expect when they go home and that they seek medical advice early should unexpected symptoms occur during the first few days after surgery.

Equipment for endoscopic surgery

Operating table

The operating table should be able to achieve the steep Trendelenberg position when needed and should also be able to be made low enough to allow comfortable use of laparoscopic instruments – in practice this is approx 10 cm lower than the height of the table for a laparotomy.

For laparoscopy, the patient should be placed in a modified lithotomy position, with minimal hip flexion so that the thighs do not obstruct the movement of laparoscopic instruments. For hysteroscopy, lithotomy position is used, with the table level or with a little head-down tilt.

Television monitors

One or more monitors are placed where the surgeon and surgeon's assistant can see them comfortably without having to turn. Introduction of high definition monitors is an important advance. The controls on a monitor are the same as those on a computer screen.

Video cameras

Cameras may either be 'single-chip' or 'three-chip'. Each coupled device in a single-chip camera is arranged in groups of three so that one will be sensitive to red, one to blue and one to green stimuli. A three-chip camera does not split the incoming light into the primary colours and each chip builds a more accurate composite picture of the colours than is possible with the single chip.

Most cameras have an automatic iris control and a manual focus. Unfortunately, the quality of the image is reduced greatly if there is a significant quantity of blood in the operative field. It is therefore important to aspirate blood to improve the view and reduce light absorption.

Light source and cable

All internal body cavities are completely dark and require high levels of illumination. The majority of laparoscopes use a 300-watt zenon light source, which is transmitted to the endoscope along a fibre-optic cable, which is vulnerable to breakage. The end of the light cable becomes very hot when used and should not be placed in direct contact with the patient or the drapes. Light is lost during transmission from the light source to the tip of the laparoscope: 7% of the available light is lost at every glass–air interface.

Electrosurgical unit

The most important method of haemostasis used during endoscopic surgery is diathermy. The generator should be capable of producing both monopolar and bipolar energy.

Hysteroscopy

The uterine cavity is a virtual cavity and requires distension with gas (CO_2) or fluid (saline or glycine) to allow visualisation with an endoscope. It requires about 40 mmHg pressure to begin to distend the uterine cavity. If bleeding occurs, this can be reduced by raising the pressure nearer to the mean arterial pressure causing a tamponade. Under local anaesthetic this may increase pain. The endometrium is supplied with an extensive network of small and large vessels which, when breached, can allow the distension medium to enter the circulation, causing gas embolus or fluid overload syndrome. This is especially a risk with operative hysteroscopy using glycine and electrosurgery. Normally at least 1 litre of glycine needs to be absorbed for a TUR syndrome to occur and results in hyponatraemia and fluid overload, sometimes leading to cerebral oedema and fits. For this reason, it is important to monitor fluid balance closely during operative hysteroscopy.

A further complication of hysteroscopy is a result of uterine perforation. This often occurs during an initial 'blind' introduction of a uterine sound or during cervical dilation rather than during hysteroscopy, which is under direct vision. Perforation may also occur during operative hysteroscopy. The possibility of damage to adjacent organs and blood vessels must be considered, with resort to laparoscopy or laparotomy if necessary.

Postoperative endometritis may be a late complication of hysteroscopy.

Equipment used for hysteroscopy

Speculum

A Sims' or Cuscoe speculum may be used to visualise the cervix. The Sims' speculum has the advantage in that it can be easy removed allowing free movement of the hysteroscopy once inserted. The cervix is often grasped with a single-tooth tenaculum or vulsellum tenaculum on the anterior lip, so as to fix the cervix during insertion of the hysteroscope and to straighten the uterine axis. It is possible, however, to perform a hysteroscopy with a no-touch technique without a speculum, starting with vaginoscopy and insertion of the hysteroscope through the cervix under direct vision. This technique is often employed for procedures performed with a small-diameter hysteroscope under local anaesthesia.

Hysteroscope

Most diagnostic hysteroscopes have a diameter between 3 mm and 5 mm. The tip may be angled (12–30 degrees) to allow visualisation into the uterine cornu, although zero-degree lenses are available and these are useful when examining the endocervix.

Hysteroscope sheath

The hysteroscope fits inside a sheath which has a channel for the inflow of distension medium. For operative hysteroscopy a larger-diameter sheath is used, with dual channels to allow inflow of distension fluid and a separate outflow of the distension fluid, together with blood. There is also a channel for operative instruments.

Fluid infusion system

Fluid has to be introduced under pressure. For diagnostic hysteroscopy, the fluid is normally a bag of saline attached via a simple infusion line. The bag is pressurised with a manual compression device set to the required pressure (40–200 mmHg). For operative hysteroscopy, a purpose-built infusion system may be used, which allows the adjustment of fluid pressure and rate of infusion to minimise fluid absorption.

Hysteroscopy procedure

1   The procedure can be performed under general or local anaesthesia.

2   Place the patient in the lithotomy position, with the buttocks slightly over the edge of the couch.

3   Perform a gentle bimanual pelvic examination to determine the size and the position of the uterus and look for any abnormal pelvic masses which were not suspected before.

4   Bladder catheterisation is generally not necessary.

5   Hysteroscopy equipment should be assembled and care taken to ensure that there are no air bubbles in the inflow system.

6   Insert a speculum to visualise the cervix.

7   Usually, no dilatation is required for diagnostic procedures, especially in the case of multiparous women.

8   The uterine cavity may first be measured with a uterine sound to check the length and the direction. If the hysteroscope will not pass easily through the cervix it is grasped by a tenaculum.

9   If dilation is required to insert the hysteroscope or allow flow of bloodstained fluid out of the uterine cavity, the dilator is introduced, only as far as the internal os, to avoid traumatising the endometrium.

10 With the distension medium running, guide the hysteroscope through the cervical canal. This should be done in stages, allowing the medium to form a microcavity in front of the optic, to allow the hysteroscope to be advanced without damage to the cervical canal.

11 Once in the uterine cavity, allow time for the distension medium to obtain a clear panoramic view.

12 Inspect every aspect of the cavity in a systematic manner, first locating both tubal ostia and lateral walls, then the anterior and posterior walls. This may be achieved by rotating the hysteroscope while keeping the camera head static (Figure 3.17).

13 Gently withdraw the hysteroscope through the cervix and study its anatomy and look for any pathology.

14 Usually, an endometrial biopsy is performed using a small metal curette or a disposable sampler.

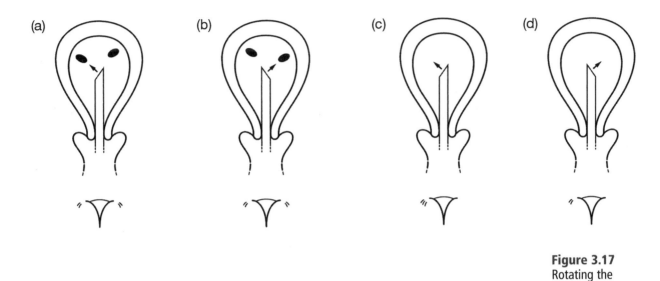

Figure 3.17
Rotating the hysteroscope

Laparoscopy

Equipment used for laparoscopy

Laparoscope

A laparoscope is simply a 5-mm or a 10-mm telescope, usually with zero- or 30-degree end viewing.

Rapid-flow insufflator

At rest, the intra-abdominal cavity is virtual and the abdominal wall lies directly on loops of bowel that rest on the major retroperitoneal blood vessels. To obtain a clear view of the contents of the abdominal cavity, it is necessary to enlarge the cavity by elevating the abdominal wall away from the underlying structures. This can be done either by upward external traction on the abdominal wall ('gasless' laparoscopy) or by distending the peritoneal cavity by filling the cavity with gas. Almost all laparoscopic surgery is performed using CO_2 gas distension technique. An insufflator is required to instil gas into the abdominal cavity under pressure. Essential features of a modern insufflator include:

■ a gauge to record the level of pressure in the intra-abdominal cavity and a system to alter the maximum desired pressure, with an automatic cut-out to prevent this level being exceeded

■ a gauge to indicate the rate of flow of gas and a system to vary the rate of flow. Early insufflators give a maximum flow rate of 3–5 litres/minute, which is insufficient. Modern insufflators deliver 9–40 litres/minute

■ a gauge to indicate the total volume of gas delivered

■ a CO_2 tank which can be replaced when empty.

Irrigation/suction system

Irrigating fluids have to be introduced into the peritoneal cavity under pressure in order to overcome the intra abdominal pressure from CO_2. Pressure is provided by using a pressure bag with a gauge wrapped around a bag of irrigating fluid (normally Hartmann's or saline solution). Suction tubing which does not collapse is attached to the wall suction via collection bottles. A more satisfactory option is to use a purpose built infusing/suction machine.

Preoperative checks

■ Ensure that the light source is fully operational and attach the camera to the laparoscope and then perform a light balance. During this procedure, the camera is taught to recognise the colour white by holding a white object (normally a surgical swab) 3 mm away from the end of the laparoscope and pressing the 'white balance' button on the camera.

■ Check the gas flow through the Verres needle. Set the pressure to a 'cut-off' of 15–20 mm of mercury with high flow. The flow of gas through the Verres needle should be approximately 1–2 litres/minute with virtually no pressure rise. Close the needle; the flow of gas should drop to zero and an alarm should sound on the machine. If there is a gas leak, the flow of gas will not drop to zero and you must check the connections and repeat the test.

■ Make sure that the diathermy plate is correctly applied.

Insertion of the primary ports

The primary ports may be inserted by a closed or opened method. Most gynaecologists favour the closed method but other surgeons usually employ the open method. Both methods are discussed. Great care must be taken when inserting laparoscopic ports in case underlying structures, particularly bowel and major blood vessels, are injured. Laparoscopy should only be undertaken where there are facilities for immediate laparotomy.

Position the patient

The patient's legs should be placed in comfortable support stirrups with slight hip flexion. The patient is level on the operating table whilst introducing a pneumo-peritoneum. After this, the patient is tilted head down.

Camera etiquette

Always keep the camera vertical – if necessary, rotate the endoscope but never the camera. Keep the tips of the operating instruments in the middle of the field of view and follow all sharp instruments in and out of the ports.

Closed entry technique for laparoscopy

Before inserting the primary trochar, the abdominal cavity needs to be distended with CO_2 gas to produce a pocket into which a sharp trochar can be inserted. This

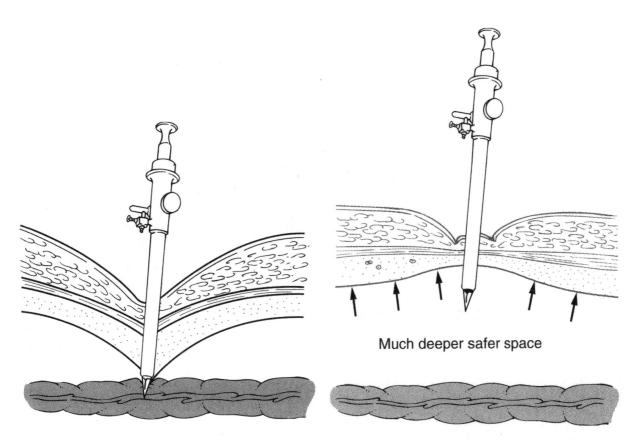

Figure 3.21 The abdominal wall is in contract with the underlying bowel

Figure 3.22 At a pressure of 15–20 mmHg a deeper space is obtained

Much deeper safer space

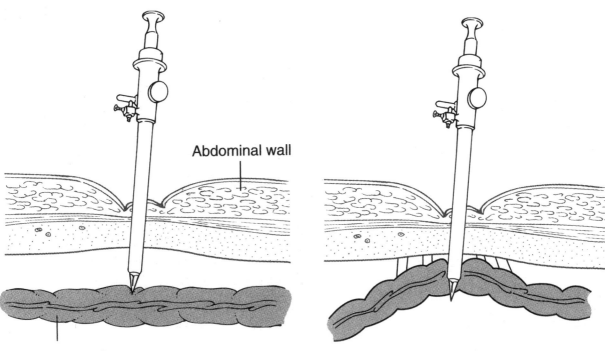

Abdominal wall

Loop of bowel

Figure 3.23 A type 1 injury

Figure 3.24 A type 2 injury

The deeper the gas bubble, the safer the subsequent trochar insertion. If a pressure of at least 15–20 mmHg (or even up to 25 mmHg) is obtained, the abdominal wall is stretched and splinted. In such circumstances, even considerable downward thrust with a trochar will not indent the abdominal wall significantly and will permit safe insertion into a substantial gas bubble (Figure 3.22). The volume of gas required to produce 20 mmHg varies between 3 litres and 12 litres but is usually around 5 litres. Once primary and secondary trochars are inserted, the pressure is returned to the standard 12–15 mmHg for the remainder of the procedure.

Insertion of the primary trochar

Insertion of the primary trochar is a potentially dangerous step, as a sharp, pointed device must be inserted through the abdominal wall without being able to see where the point is going. Damage to bowel and the major blood vessels is a particular concern. The type of entry related injury may be classified into type 1 injuries, which are produced to abdominal contents located in the normal positions (Figure 3.23) and type 2 injuries, which are produced in abnormally located structures (Figure 3.24).

Type 2 injuries may be anticipated from the patient's history. The most common type 2 lesion is bowel adherent to the abdominal wall under the entry site. This is much more likely to occur in those who have had previous intra-abdominal surgery, particularly if it was a midline incision, and extra care must be taken.

Bowel adherent to the umbilicus may be detected by a carefully performed Palmer's aspiration test. If this test is positive, an alternative entry site should be chosen.

Steps for primary trochar insertion (closed entry)

1. Lie the patient flat.

2. Choose a trochar which can be 'palmed' to prevent uncontrolled deep entry.

3. Insert the trochar vertically through the base of the umbilicus.

4. As soon as cavity is entered, withdraw the sharp trochar and advance towards the pelvis (disposable trochars may be spring loaded).

5. Insert the laparoscope and perform an immediate 360-degree inspection to ensure that there is no adherent or damaged bowel and no retroperitoneal bleeding.

   The careful use of this recommended technique should allow type 1 injuries to be avoided by entering the abdomen in the safety zone of the large gas bubble and should allow the prevention of most type 2 injuries.

Open entry for laparoscopy

In an attempt to avoid the risk associated with closed laparoscopy, the technique of open laparoscopy was developed by Harrith Hasson, a gynaecologist from Chicago, USA. With this technique, a mini-laparotomy incision is made just below the umbilicus and a blunt-ended trochar inserted under direct vision into the cavity. A modification of the Hasson method is as follows.

Steps for open laparoscopy

1. Make either a 2 cm vertical incision (extending the primary failed entry incision) in the umbilical skin or transverse subumbilical incision down to the fascia.

2. Clean and elevate the fascia with forceps and incise vertically or transversely.

3. A stay suture may be inserted into sheath either side of the incision.

4. Enter the peritoneum with blunt-ended forceps or by picking up with a tissue forceps and incising.

5. Carefully insert a blunt-ended trochar.

6. If the trochar is not airtight, secure with stay sutures and 'cone' to produce a seal.

   This approach has been widely used, particularly by non-gynaecological surgeons. There is no evidence that it reduces entry injuries but it is likely that any such complication can be diagnosed immediately and repaired.

Alternative entry site

When periumbilical adhesions are suspected, an alternative primary entry site should be selected. In the absence of previous upper abdominal surgery, the area of the abdomen with the lowest risk of abdominal wall adhesions is the left hypochondrium. The Palmer's entry point is 3 cm beneath the ninth rib in the midclavicular line. Closed entry in this site is achieved using the same technique described above via the umbilicus.

Insertion of secondary ports

In all operative and most diagnostic laparoscopies, one or more ports are needed for instruments to be passed into the abdominal cavity. In gynaecological surgery, almost all of these ports are inserted below the umbilicus. The most important structures in the abdominal wall to avoid are the inferior and superficial epigastric vessels.

In most women, these structures can be identified by a combination of direct laparoscopic visualisation and transillumination. Transillumination alone is often inadequate because, except in women who are thin, the inferior epigastric vessels lie beneath the recti muscles. Transillumination often identifies the superficial vessels and so should be performed simultaneously with direct laparoscopic visualisation.

Secondary trochars should be inserted, either in the relatively avascular midline or lateral to the course of the inferior epigastric vessels, taking care to avoid the superficial epigastric vessels.

Laparoscopic exit techniques

Care should be taken when removing the ports. Each of the secondary ports should be carefully removed under direct laparoscopic vision and the sites inspected for intra-abdominal bleeding.

The laparoscope is removed slowly, using the opportunity to make a final inspection of the abdominal contents adjacent to the end of the primary port. The final step in the exit technique should be to remove the primary port. Open the valve and allow

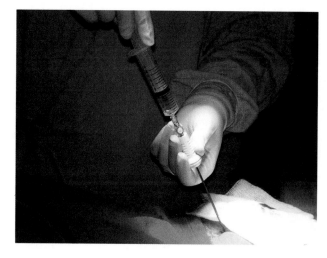

Figure 3.25 Withdrawing fluid

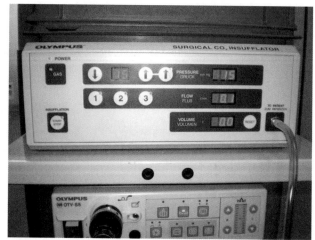

Figure 3.26 The insufflator

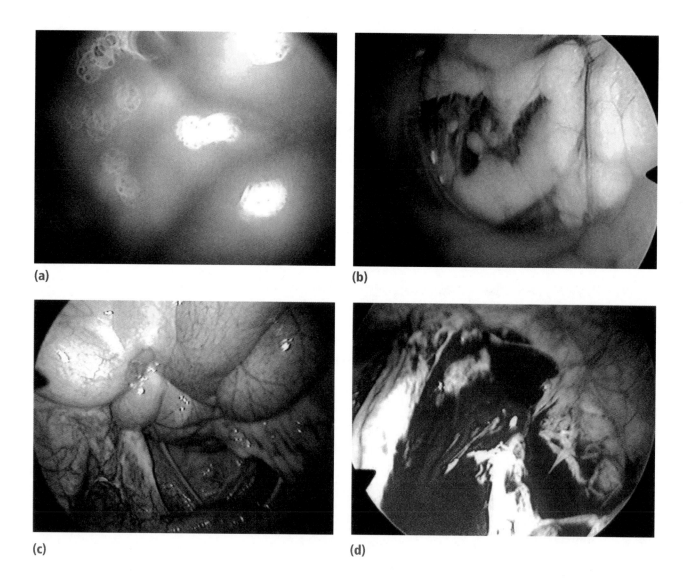

(a)

(b)

(c)

(d)

Figure 3.27 Your first view of the abdominal cavity

the CO_2 to escape then withdraw the port with the valve still open. This technique should minimise the risk of bowel or omentum being sucked into the end of the port.

Each wound should be repaired. Small (5 mm) incisions will usually only require a single-layer skin closure. Small (7–8 mm) suprapubic incisions, which are often used during female sterilisation, appear to be at low risk of subsequent hernia formation and are also often only closed with a skin suture. Other incisions require closure of underlying fascia to prevent hernia formation of wound dehiscence. Lateral incisions greater than 5 mm should be repaired in layers, taking great care to suture the rectus sheath. In many cases, adequate external visualisation and access to the sheath will not be possible because of the small size of the incision. In these circumstances, closure with a J-shaped needle or special port-closure device is necessary.

Closure of the umbilical incision must include closure of the umbilical fascia and rectus sheath if the incision is extended or subumbilical. This may be sufficient but a skin suture may also be required.

Suggested reading

Royal College of Obstetricians and Gynaecologists. *Diagnostic Hysteroscopy under General Anaesthesia.* Consent Advice 1. London: RCOG; 2004.

Royal College of Obstetricians and Gynaecologists. *Diagnostic Laparoscopy.* Consent Advice 2. London: RCOG; 2004.

Laparoscopy scenario

The following scenario is intended to be used as part of a group session to stimulate discussion around laparoscopy and its likely pitfalls.

Closed laparoscopic entry and optimisation of equipment

1. You are about to undertake a diagnostic laparoscopy. The patient is anaesthetised and draped ready to start. First you want to test the insufflator but find that there is no gas flow.

   Consider the possible reasons for this.

2. You insert an umbilical Veress needle and undertake a saline (Palmer's) test. After injecting saline you then withdraw fluid (Figure 3.25).

   Consider the possible reasons for this.

3. You reinsert the needle directly via the umbilicus, feeling for a 'double click' and test before you ask for the insufflator to be turned on. Initially, there is an insufflation (intra-abdominal) pressure of greater than 10 mmHg (Figure 3.26).

   Consider the causes.

4. Insufflation is achieved at low pressure (5–8 mmHg), you ask for high-flow insufflation after 1 litre of CO_2 and finally reach 20 mmHg after 4.5 litres of CO_2. You remove the Veress needle. Using a guarded method, you place a 10 mm trochar through your umbilical incision and insert the laparoscope with the camera attached. You look at the monitor and notice the monitor screen is blank.

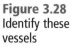

Figure 3.28
Identify these
vessels

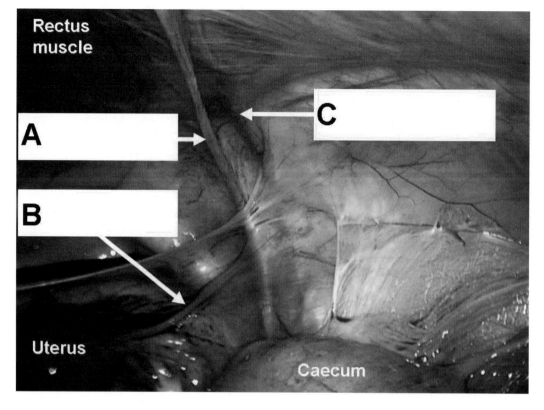

What are the likely causes?

5. You have a view down the laparoscope but the screen appears dark.

   Consider the possible causes.

6. The camera is attached but the image is very blurred so that intra-abdominal structures can not be identified (Figure 3.27a).

   Consider the possible reasons for this.

7. When you first look at a clear view through the laparoscope, it appears that the tip is surrounded by fat with no other structures visible (Figure 3.27b).

   Consider the reasons for this.

8. Your first view of the abdominal cavity is unusual (Figure 3.27c).

   Consider what is being seen.

9. Despite introduction of a secondary port on the left side of the abdomen and a probe to manipulate the bowel, it is not possible to get a clear view of the pelvis or the pouch or Douglas (the cul de sac between the rectum and vagina).

   What are the possible causes?

10. You notice a significant amount of blood that was not present initially (Figure 3.27d).

    Consider the possibilities and what you would do for each one.

11. Identify the positions of the round ligament, inferior epigastric vessels and obliterated umbilical vessels in Figure 3.28.

Checklist for laparoscopy scenario

Closed laparoscopy entry and optimisation of equipment

1. No gas flow

- ■ Veress needle blocked or tap turned off
- ■ Insufflator not turned on
- ■ Insufflation tubing not connected
- ■ Insufflation tubing kinked or blocked
- ■ Gas tank not turned on or empty CO$_2$ tank

Scenario: The camera stack wheel is compressing the insufflation tube and is moved so that your test is now satisfactory.

2. Fluid withdrawn

- ■ Veress needle in abdominal wall (preperitoneal)
- ■ Veress needle in omentum or other intra-abdominal structure
- ■ Intra-abdominal fluid/ascites
- ■ Ovarian cyst perforated by Veress needle
- ■ Full bladder perforated by Veress needle

Scenario: The fluid is clear, with no blood or faeces and it is not discoloured. The Veress needle had been inserted subumbilically; it likely that the needle tip is lying in the preperitoneal fat of the abdominal wall.

3. Insufflation pressure of greater than 10 mmHg

- ■ Veress needle tap not fully turned on
- ■ Insufflation tubing kinked or blocked
- ■ Insufflator initially set to high flow (35 litres/minute) rather than low flow (1 litre/minute)
- ■ Veress needle in abdominal wall/preperitoneal fat
- ■ Veress needle in bowel/omentum

Scenario: You have accidentally turned the Veress needle tap off slightly while inserting it. By opening the tap fully, the pressure reduces to 5 mmHg insufflation (intra-abdominal) pressure.

4. The monitor screen is blank

- ■ Monitor or camera stack not connected or turned on
- ■ Monitor or stack broken
- ■ Light source or lead not connected or turned on
- ■ Light source bulb broken

Scenario: The lead from the camera head is not plugged into the camera stack. Once it is plugged in, the screen flickers and gives a view.

5. The screen appears dark

- Bright overhead theatre lights still on
- Light lead not fully connected to light source
- Damaged light lead
- Light source on manual and set to low rather than automatic light setting

Scenario: The light cable was not fully engaged with the light source. Once you rectify this, the screen has a bright image (note: a haemoperitoneum can also give a dark view due to light absorption by blood).

6. The image is very blurred

- Camera head out of focus
- Laparoscope tip soiled (blood or pus) or condensation
- Condensation between laparoscope eyepiece and camera head
- Damaged laparoscope or camera system

Scenario: The laparoscope tip is soiled with blood; after removing it and wiping the tip, a clear view is obtained (note: diathermy created smoke or vapour may also reduce visibility during surgery).

7. Tip is surrounded by fat with no other structures visible

- Primary port not fully inserted (preperitoneal fat)
- Laparoscope or port tip buried in omentum/other structure

Scenario: As you withdraw the laparoscope, the omentum falls off the tip. On direct vision, there does not appear to be any significant trauma to the omentum.

8. View of the abdominal cavity is unusual

- The camera head is not orientated correctly, so that the abdomen appears upside down

Scenario: By rotation of the camera head on the laparoscope eyepiece, the abdominal cavity is orientated properly so that you can proceed.

9. Not possible to get a clear view of the pelvis or the pouch or Douglas

- Insufficient head down (Trendelenberg) tilt so that bowel is obscuring the pelvis
- Pelvic pathology (endometriotic or other adhesions) obscuring view
- Uterus not anteverted adequately
- Inadequate pneumoperitoneum (loss of gas, insufflator not turned on or disconnected)

Scenario: The anaesthetist has already given a head-down tilt but is happy to increase this. There is still not a good view, even after manoeuvring the small bowel away from the pelvis and adjusting the uterine manipulator to get maximum anteversion. The insufflation tubing has become detached and reconnection results in a good proper pneumoperitoneum so that a good view is obtained.

10. A significant amount of blood

- ■ Damage to inferior epigastric vessels
- ■ Bleeding from primary port site
- ■ Bleeding from elsewhere in abdomen (e.g. iliac vessels, omental injury)

Scenario: On direct inspection, fairly persistent bleeding is coming directly from the site of the secondary port; it appears that the inferior epigastric artery has been damaged. You can secure haemostasis through the incision with a suture and J-shaped needle (alternatives could be bipolar cautery or an endoscopic closure method but with a plan to convert to open surgical haemostasis if this is not successful).

11. Identify the positions of the round ligament, inferior epigastric vessels and obliterated umbilical vessels

- ■ A = Obliterated umbilical vessels
- ■ B = Round ligament
- ■ C = Internal markings of inferior epigastric vessels